OTOSCOPY

a structured approach

OTOSCOPY

a structured approach

P J WORMALD FCS (SA) FRCS
Consultant Surgeon, ENT Department,
Groote Schuur Hospital, Cape Town, South Africa

G G BROWNING MD FRCS
Professor of Otolaryngology, and Consultant in Administrative Charge,
Department of Otolaryngology, University of Glasgow,
and Senior Consultant Otologist, British MRC Institute of Hearing Research,
Scottish Section, Glasgow Royal Infirmary,
Glasgow, United Kingdom

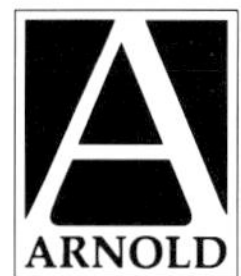

A member of the Hodder Headline Group
LONDON • SYDNEY • AUCKLAND

First published in Great Britain 1996 by
Arnold, a member of the Hodder Headline Group,
338 Euston Road, London NW1 3BH

Whilst the advice and information in this book is believed to be true and
accurate at the date of going to press, neither the authors nor the publisher
can accept any legal responsibility or liability for any errors or omissions
that may be made. In particular (but without limiting the generality of the
preceding disclaimer) every effort has been made to check drug dosages;
however it is still possible that errors have been missed. Furthermore,
dosage schedules are constantly being revised and new side-effects
recognized. For these reasons the reader is strongly urged to consult the
drug companies' printed instructions before administering any of the drugs
recommended in this book.

British Library Cataloguing in Publication Data
A catalogue record for this book is available from the British Library

Library of Congress Cataloguing-in-Publication Data
A catalog record for this book is available from the Library of Congress

ISBN 0 340 613769 (pb)

Typeset in 10/12pt New Baskerville by Scribe Design
Printed and bound in Hong Kong

CONTENTS

Preface — vii

Acknowledgements — viii

CHAPTER 1 — General principles of structured otoscopy — 1

CHAPTER 2 — The normal ear — 3

CHAPTER 3 — More common otoscopic diagnoses — 10

CHAPTER 4 — Hearing impairment in adults — 17

CHAPTER 5 — Hearing impairment in children — 29

CHAPTER 6 — The painful ear — 42

CHAPTER 7 — The discharging ear — 52

CHAPTER 8 — Ear trauma — 75

CHAPTER 9 — Techniques of examination — 78

References — 89

Index — 91

To Fiona, Nicholas and Sarah
PJW

To all those whom I have loved and have loved in return
GGB

PREFACE

Changes in medicine take place slowly but this seems particularly to apply to its teaching. Little has changed since the introduction of glass lantern slides, apart from the topics being taught and the times allocated to them. Innovations there have been, but they have been technical ones which make conventional presentations easier, a recent example being computerised slide production. Even then, innovations such as videos are primarily used to ease the lecture workload and to instruct on patients to a larger audience rather than being used to teach in a novel way.

We hope this text uses improved technology to teach otology in a novel way. The improved technology is the rod telescope used to photograph the ear, along with the ability to reproduce the resultant photographs more cheaply. The novel teaching method is the structured approach: we begin with the situations from which otologists start to reach a diagnosis; we then show how otoscopy can take readers along the stages in a decision tree to arrive at a diagnosis. This approach is deductive and allows trainees to stop at whatever level of competence they wish to achieve.

The stimulus for a change in teaching methods comes from many sources but not, contrary to what is commonly thought, from revamping the curriculum. This usually results in a rehash of the existing course with more topics being added and nothing being deleted. Changes should start by defining the aims of instruction. This is where an academic department has an advantage as it is usually a meeting place of thinkers from different disciplines and countries. The concepts of otoscopy, as elucidated here, have evolved over the years at Glasgow Royal Infirmary. In this, Stuart Gatehouse and Ken Robinson, as audiological scientists, and Iain Swan, as an otologist, have been particularly influential.

PJ Wormald joined the group from South Africa for a period in 1993 and questioned whether the teaching of otoscopy could not be improved. When looked at scientifically, it became obvious that postgraduates in otolaryngology were not proficient in otoscopy without training (Wormald *et al.*, 1995). Whilst there is a difference between coming to a diagnosis from a photograph and in a patient, it seemed sensible to teach otoscopy initially from photographs. Hence the development of our structured approach to otoscopy.

The production of this book has been a collaborative process. PJW took over 95% of the photographs. Grant Bates and Iain RC Swan contributed the remainder. Again, while PJW drew the majority of the illustrations, Figures 2.1, 2.2, 2.8, 4.10, 5.30, 7.8a and b, 9.1 and 9.2 are reproduced with permission from Butterworth-Heinemann Ltd. GGB wrote the final text but was considerably guided in this by PJW. At various stages Chris Prescott, Iain RC Swan and Daniel S Morrison gave helpful comments. Finally there are many medical undergraduates and postgraduates in Glasgow, Oxford and Cape Town who have helped us to understand the difficulties that beginners have with otoscopy and enabled us to modify our method.

PJW GGB 1995

ACKNOWLEDGEMENTS

The authors and publisher would like to thank the following for permission to use copyright material in this book:

Butterworth for figure 2.8 from Browning, G.G., *Clinical Audiology and Otology* (1986); and for figure 4.10 from Browning G.G., 'Pathology of inflammatory conditions of the external and middle ear' in *Scott-Brown's Otolaryngology*, 5th Edn, Otology Volume (1987) edited by A.G. Kerr and J.B. Booth; Butterworth-Heinemann for figures 2.1, 7.8a and b, 9.1 and 9.2, from Browning, G.G., *Updated ENT*, 3rd Edn (1994), and for figures 2.2 and 5.30 from Browning, G.G., 'Aetiopathology of inflammatory conditions of the external and middle ear' in *Scott-Brown's Otolaryngology*, 6th Edn, Otology Volume (1995) edited by J.B. Booth.

CHAPTER 1

GENERAL PRINCIPLES OF A STRUCTURED APPROACH TO OTOSCOPY

Otoscopy is a skill that can be difficult to master. It is an important skill to acquire for those involved in managing patients with ear complaints, as external and middle ear conditions are almost invariably diagnosed on otoscopy. The level of skill required depends on what action the otoscopist is going to take as a result of the findings. A basic level is required by audiometricians and hearing aid dispensers to distinguish diseased from non-diseased ears so that they can refer the former on. A greater degree of skill is required by primary care physicians, such as general practitioners in the United Kingdom and paediatricians in the United States and Europe, as they not only need to distinguish diseased from non-diseased ears, but also to recognise some conditions, such as acute otitis media, which are primarily treated by them. Finally, the highest degree of skill is required by otolaryngologists who often have to make subtle judgements – usually surgical ones – on their otoscopic findings, frequently aided by the use of a microscope.

BASIC AND SPECIALIST SECTIONS

Each section of this text starts with the basic information required by all otoscopists. This is followed, where appropriate, by a specialist section. Whilst non-specialists may wish to increase their diagnostic abilities by going through the specialist sections, they should expect these sections to be more difficult to put into practice, particularly if they do not have specialist equipment, such as suction and a microscope, to help them.

A STRUCTURED APPROACH

The time honoured way to learn otoscopy is by an apprenticeship system whereby it is expected that if a large number of ears are seen, the pupil will automatically learn what is wrong with them. The classic scenario is for a tutor to ask the pupil 'Do you see that?' without explaining what 'that' is. The pupil can only respond by saying 'Yes', otherwise they make themselves, or even worse their tutor, seem stupid. That such an apprenticeship method is weak is evident to all when trainees' abilities are more formally tested in examination circumstances.

When skilled otoscopists are asked how they assess an ear, they usually admit to having a series of questions that they ask themselves. The sequence in which they do this varies between otologists but most often the questions are posed in a structured manner depending on the patient's symptoms. There is no reason why such a structured approach cannot be taught. It is recognised that this requires decision trees with which many clinicians find themselves uncomfortable. Decision trees are often seen as a scientist's approach to common sense, but common sense has to be learned and a structured approach can make this easier. As might be expected, the order in which questions are asked in the decision tree varies between examiners and from case to case. However, the questions themselves do not vary.

Look at summary tree 1.1

In this text at the beginning of each symptom-based chapter there is a decision tree that summarises the questions that should be posed and the routes to the final diagnoses for that specific symptom. To make the understanding of each branch of the tree easier, in some chapters it is broken into alphabetical branches which are reproduced thereafter. To make their understanding easier, questions are in italics, and the final diagnosis is in bold. The circled numbers at various points allow correlation with the text.

SYMPTOM-BASED APPROACH

Many texts use a disease-based approach which, though informative, is less valuable to a practising clinician than is a symptom-based approach. The latter is used here though it is recognised that, to facilitate this, the various diseases need to be defined. Chapter 3 gives a brief explanation of the more common otological conditions which will make the understanding of the symptom-based chapters easier. Some conditions have multiple symptoms and are thus mentioned in several chapters. However, to prevent duplication each condition is only fully discussed under its most common presenting symptom.

Most textbooks on otoscopy start with a technique section. This section is important but, as most would not consider this particularly

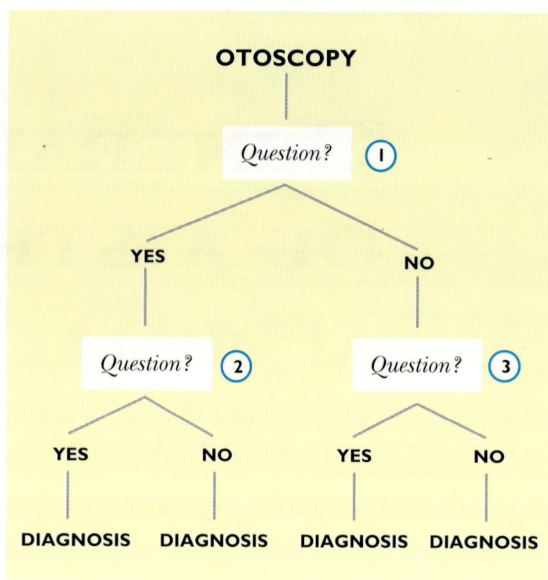

Summary tree 1.1 Layout of decision trees.

difficult, it appears in this text in the last chapter. The techniques of clearing the external auditory canal of wax, debris and pus are included in this chapter to avoid unnecessary repetition of the statement that 'the first thing to do is to clear the external canal so that a good view is obtained'.

THE PHOTOGRAPHS

In this text the ear photographs have been taken with a rod telescope. This gives a wide-angled view, which is superior to that obtained via an aural speculum (pages 80–81). Hence readers will often find that when they perform otoscopy with an otoscope it is difficult to obtain as good a view of the tympanic membrane as might be expected from the illustrations in this text. This should not dispirit them but encourage them to continue to practise. In particular, they should learn to alter the angle of the otoscope to view different areas of the ear.

CHAPTER 2

THE NORMAL EAR

Classically the ear is divided into the external, middle and inner ears (Figure 2.1), the first terminating at the tympanic membrane, which is considered part of the middle ear. After clearance of any visually obstructing wax, debris or pus, otoscopy usually allows the external ear and tympanic membrane to be examined. The tympanic membrane is usually altered by middle ear disease. As a consequence, most diseases of the external and middle ear are diagnosed by otoscopy and the success or otherwise of management is monitored by repeat otoscopy.

Look at summary tree 2.1

Otoscopy requires recognition of whether the external ear canal and tympanic membrane are within the range of normal. The decision tree summarises the stages of otoscopy which distinguish diseased from normal ears. The external auditory canal is first examined ①. The tympanic membrane is then identified and its two component parts, the pars tensa ② and the pars flaccida ③, are examined for normality.

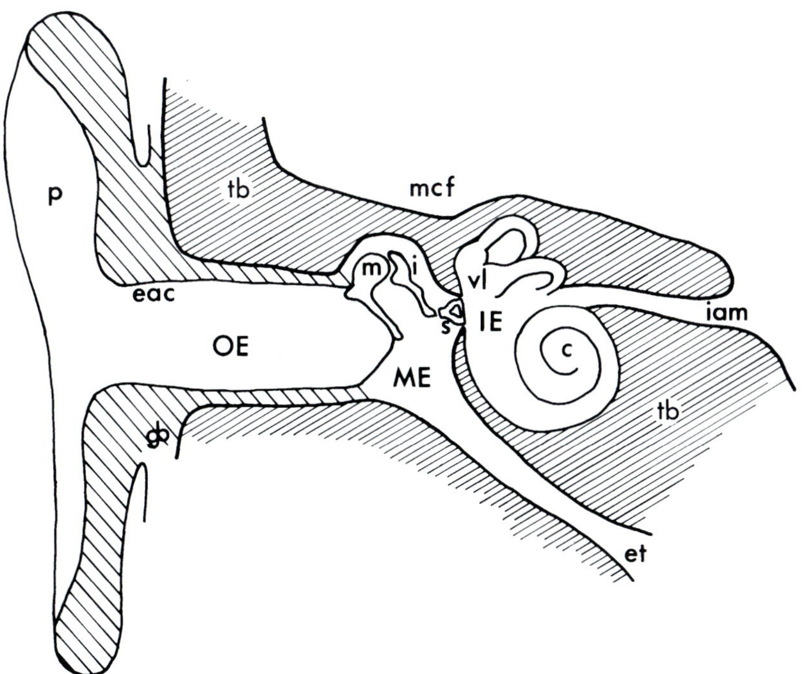

FIGURE 2.1 *Coronal section through the right ear, seen from the front. Note in particular the three main parts, the outer, the middle and the inner ear. OE, outer ear; ME, middle ear; IE, inner ear; p, pinna; eac, external auditory canal; m, malleus; i, incus; s, stapes; vl, vestibular labyrinth; c, cochlea; tb, temporal bone; mcf, middle cranial fossa; iam, internal auditory meatus; et, Eustachian tube.*

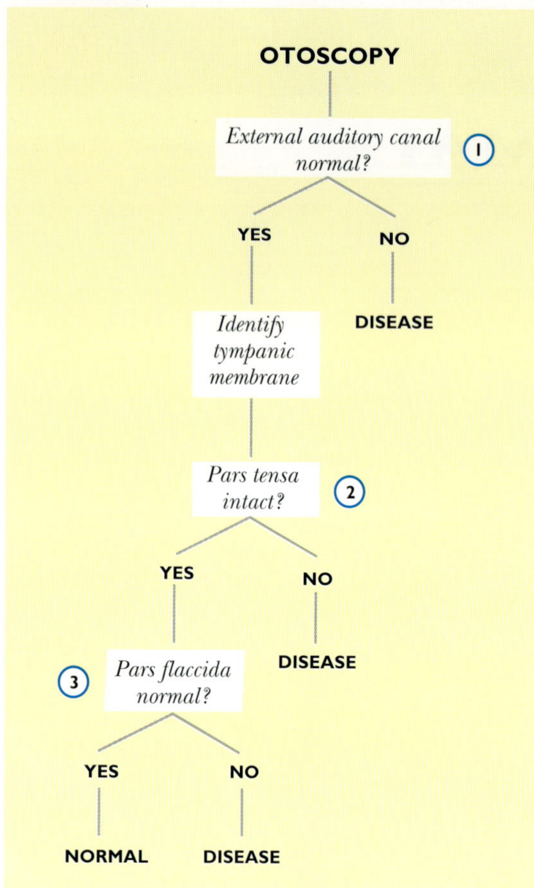

Summary tree 2.1 Steps in otoscopy.

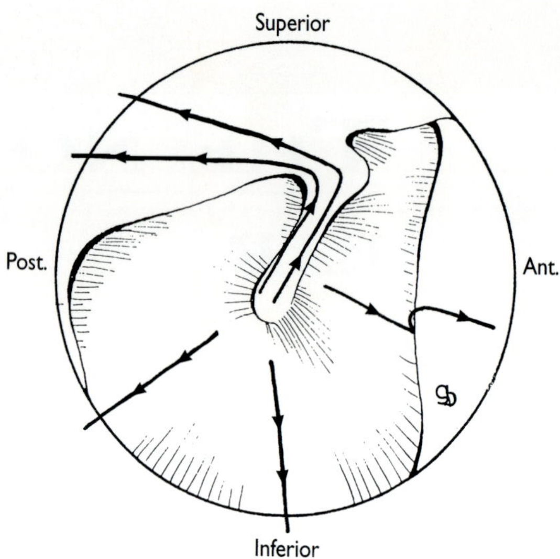

FIGURE 2.2 *Routes of migration of epithelium of the tympanic membrane to the canal wall.*

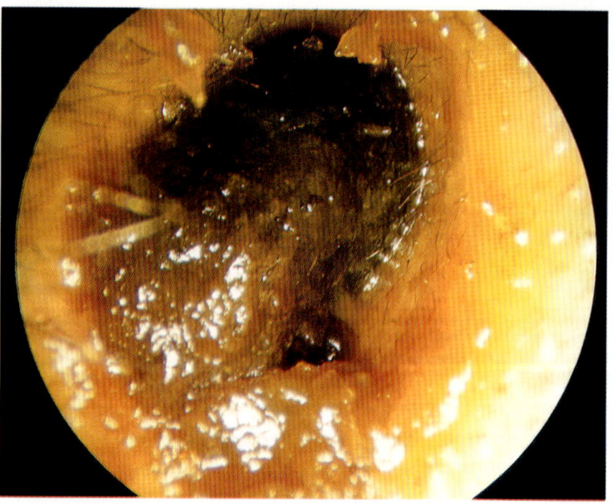

FIGURE 2.3 *Wax debris in right ear. Note the enmeshed hairs which are common.*

EXTERNAL AUDITORY CANAL

The external auditory canal is lined by skin (keratinised squamous epithelium) which in addition to having hair follicles has specialised wax (cerumen) secreting glands in its outer third. As elsewhere, the skin sheds squames but to prevent these building up in the canal, the squamous epithelium gradually migrates from the tympanic membrane out the canal. Figure 2.2 shows the standard route of migration from the tympanic membrane to the canal, this having been worked out by sequentially photographing ink dots. Wax is shed along with the squames.

Q *Is the external auditory canal normal?* ①

The most common abnormality of the external canal is wax retention (Figure 2.3). The reasons why this occurs are uncertain but the misguided use of cotton buds to clean out the ear does not help. The mould of a hearing aid also tends to push wax back into the canal. When wax is impacted against the tympanic membrane (Figure 2.4), a hearing impairment will result

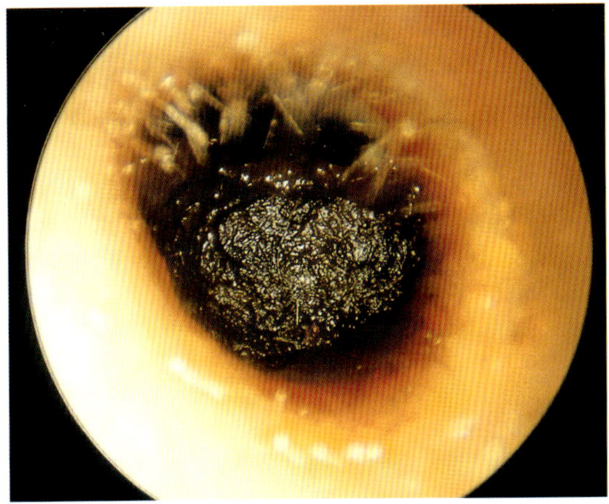

FIGURE 2.4 *Wax impacted against left tympanic membrane. Note wax indentation due to cotton bud.*

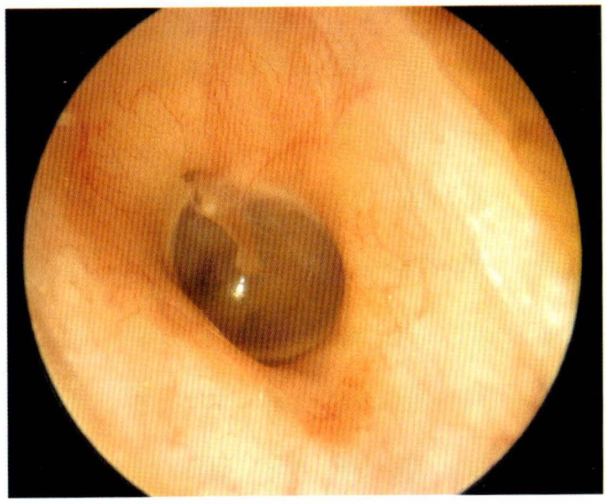

FIGURE 2.5 *Normal skin in the left external auditory canal.*

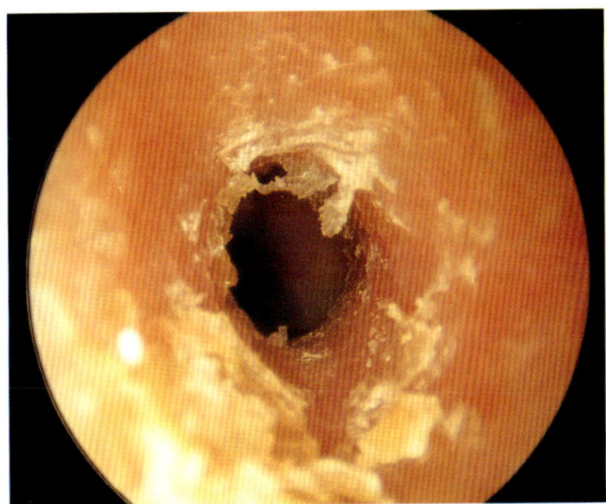

FIGURE 2.6 *Otitis externa (left). Red, swollen and oedematous canal skin.*

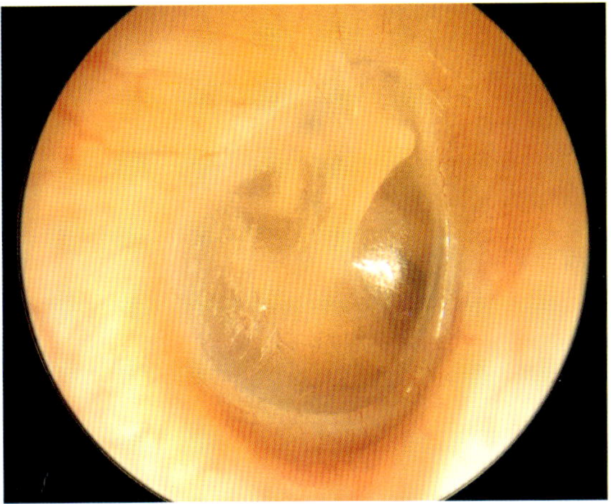

(a)

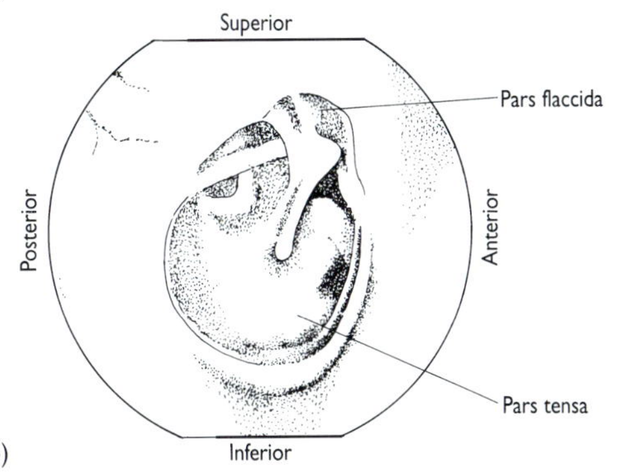

(b)

FIGURE 2.7a and b *Normal right tympanic membrane illustrating pars tensa and pars flaccida.*

but this degree of impaction is relatively uncommon (Chapter 9). The most common reason to remove wax is to visualise the canal and tympanic membrane.

Normally the canal skin (Figure 2.5) looks like skin anywhere else on the body. When inflamed, it first becomes red, then progressively it becomes more swollen and indurated (Figure 2.6). A secondary, inflammatory exudate is common.

THE TYMPANIC MEMBRANE: THE PARS TENSA AND PARS FLACCIDA

The tympanic membrane is divided into the pars tensa and the pars flaccida (Schrapnell's membrane) (Figure 2.7). Histologically, both have three layers, an outer squamous epithelial, a middle fibrous and an inner flat mucosal layer. The pars tensa is the larger inferior portion whose fibrous layer is directionally organised (Figure 2.8). There are radial fibres which are attached to the malleus handle. There are circumferential fibres which are more abundant at the periphery and concentrated posteriorly, inferiorly and anteriorly, but not superiorly in a fibrous annulus. Anatomically the anterior and posterior malleolar ligaments separate the pars tensa from the pars flaccida but these are not usually identified unless the tympanic membrane is retracted. The pars flaccida is thus in the superior part of the middle ear or the attic. The fibrous layer in the pars flaccida is not directionally organised.

The majority of middle ear diseases affect the pars tensa, and this is the part that is usually initially assessed on otoscopy. Isolated disease of the pars flaccida is less common but important to recognise (pages 40–41).

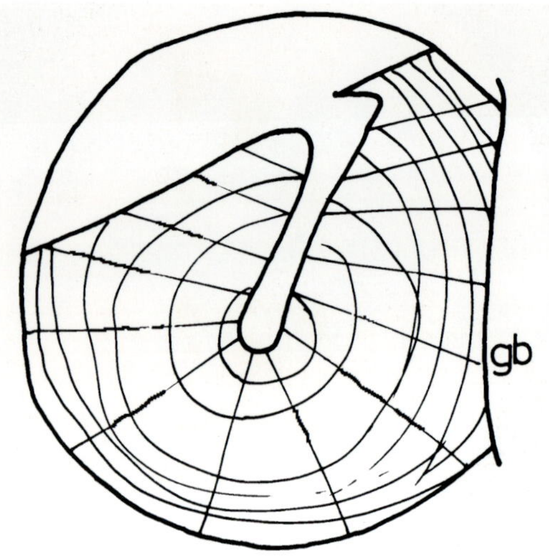

FIGURE 2.8 *Drawing to illustrate the direction of fibrous tissue in the pars tensa. Right ear.*

Q *Is the tympanic membrane normal?* ② ③

The inexperienced otoscopist frequently does not angle the speculum anteriorly enough and can find it difficult to identify the tympanic membrane. The key is to identify the handle of the malleus. If the malleus cannot be found after looking in all directions and the canal is visually clear, then the tympanic membrane is

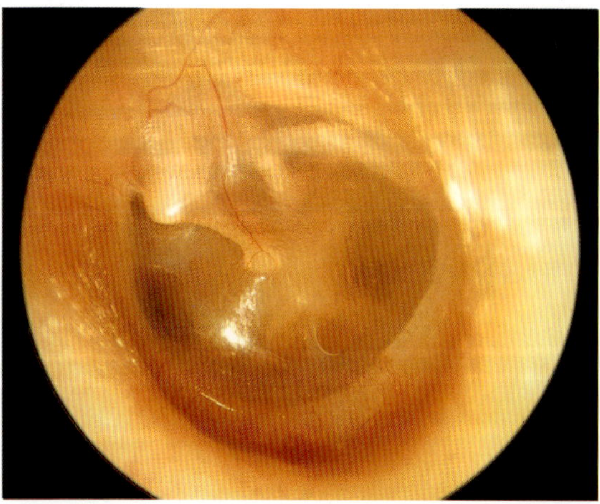

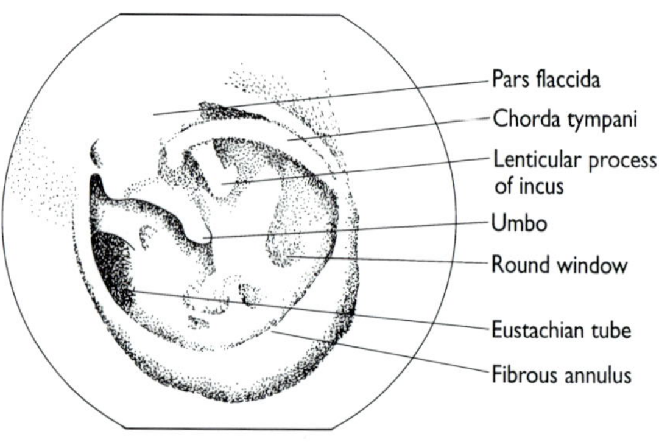

FIGURE 2.9a and b *Normal left tympanic membrane. Drawing illustrates important middle ear anatomy structures often identified behind the tympanic membrane.*

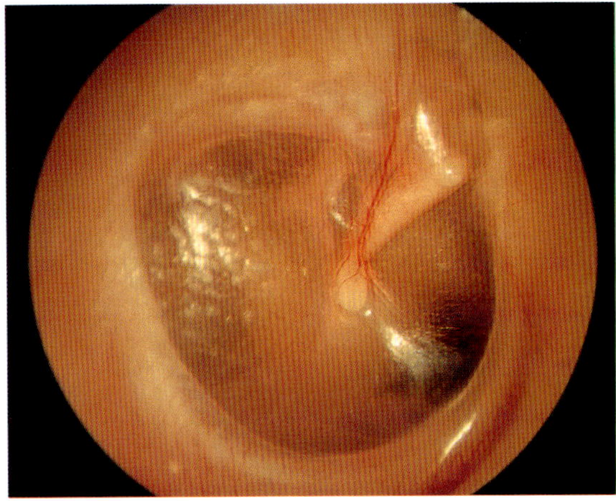

FIGURE 2.10 *Normal right tympanic membrane. More marked vasculature over malleus handle but within the normal range.*

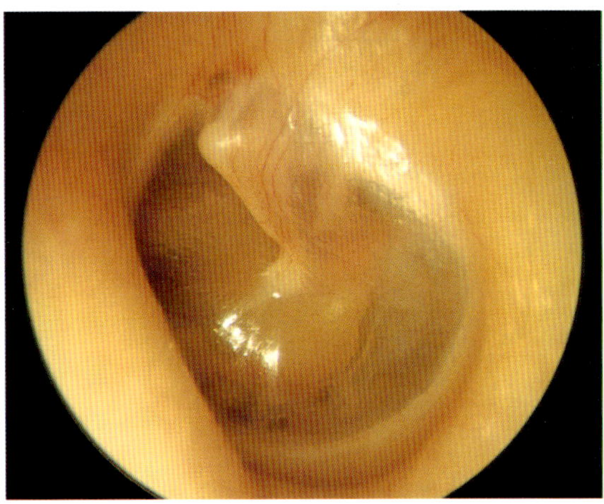

FIGURE 2.11 *Normal left tympanic membrane. Anterior pars tensa not entirely visible due to anterior canal bulge of temporomandibular joint.*

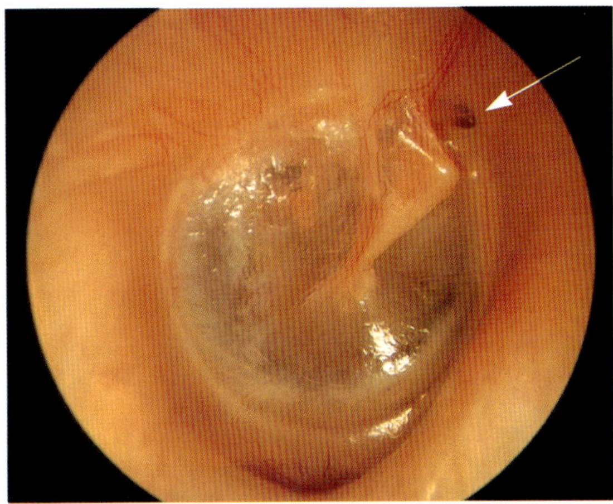

FIGURE 2.12 *Normal right tympanic membrane. Pars tensa slightly opacified especially at periphery. Pars flaccida more dimpled (arrowed) than previous illustrations.*

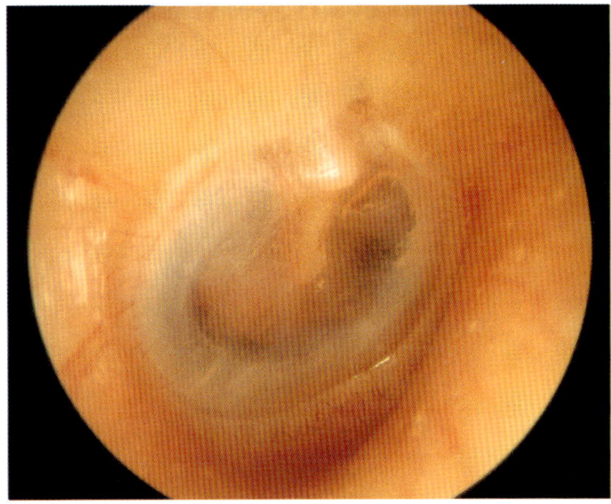

FIGURE 2.13 *Normal left tympanic membrane. Pars tensa opaque. This is sometimes associated with ageing.*

abnormal. What the abnormality is will be dealt with later. If found, it should be possible to identify the pars tensa and pars flaccida and decide whether they are normal or not.

This question is most easily answered by three further questions. First ask the question '*Are the pars tensa and flaccida intact?*', then '*Are they normal in position?*', and '*Are they of a normal consistency and colour?*'. If at any stage the answer is no, then there is disease.

Figures 2.9 to 2.14 are a range of normal tympanic membranes illustrating the minor variations in anatomy, consistency, colour and degree of vasculature. In each illustration the answer to the three questions given above is 'Yes'.

Q   Is the pars tensa intact? ②

Figure 2.15 is an example where the answer to the question '*Is the pars tensa intact?*' is 'No'.

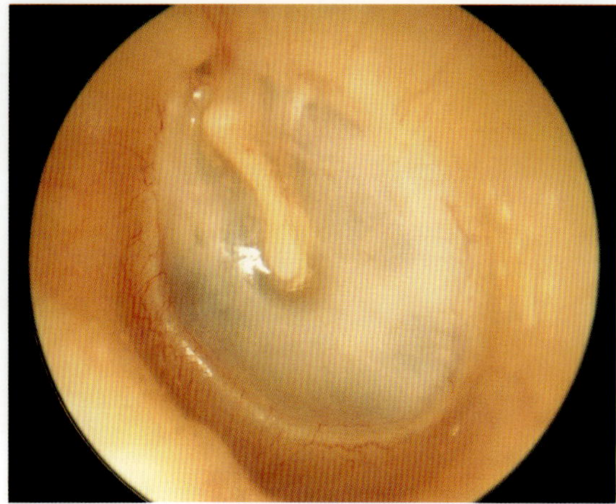

FIGURE 2.14 *Normal left tympanic membrane. Very opaque pars tensa. Pars flaccida dimpled.*

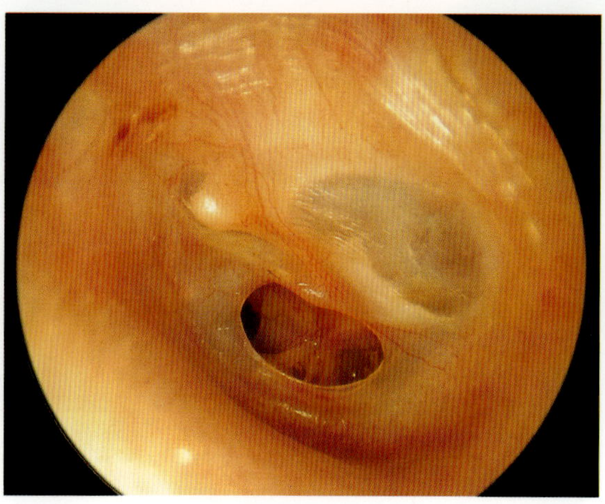

FIGURE 2.15 *Pars tensa defect of left chronic otitis media.*

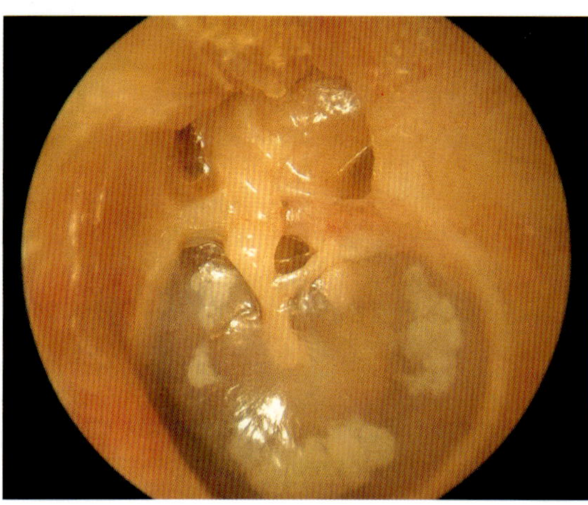

FIGURE 2.16 *Pars flaccida defect associated with left chronic otitis media.*

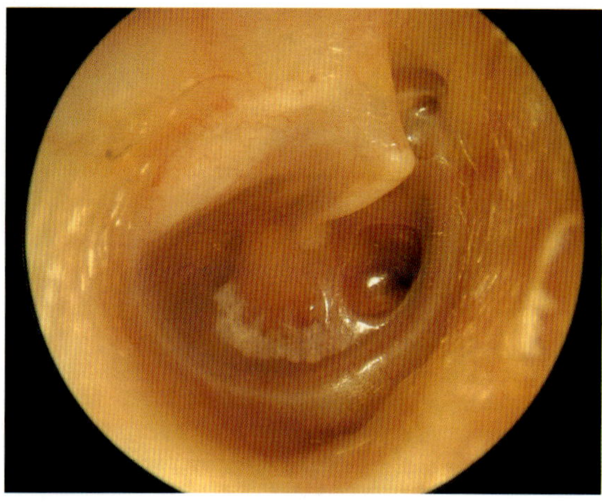

FIGURE 2.17 *Pars tensa and pars flaccida retraction associated with right otitis media with effusion.*

There is a defect or perforation through which a view of the middle ear can be obtained.

Figure 2.16 is an example where the answer to the question '*Is the pars flaccida intact?*' is 'No'. When the pars tensa or flaccida are not intact the most likely diagnosis is **chronic (suppurative) otitis media**.

When the pars tensa and flaccida are intact the next question is '*Are they in a normal position?*'.

Q Are the pars tensa and flaccida in a normal position?

The most common abnormality of position is retraction. Figure 2.17 is an example where the pars tensa and the pars flaccida are both retracted but still intact. The most likely diagnosis in such ears is **otitis media with effusion**.

When the pars tensa and flaccida are intact and in a normal position the next question is '*Are they of a normal consistency and colour?*'.

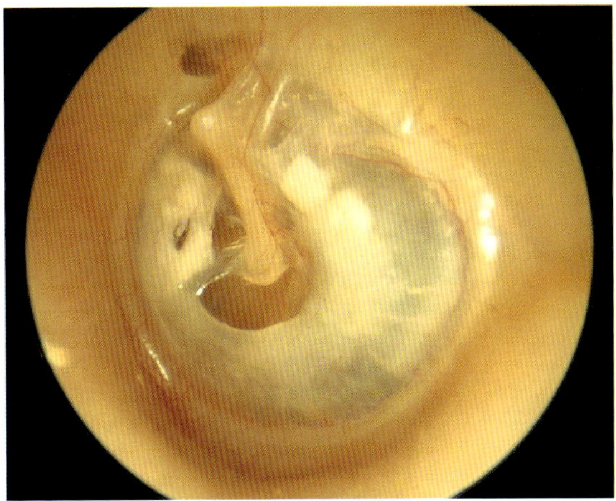

FIGURE 2.18 *Scarred pars tensa associated with left healed otitis media.*

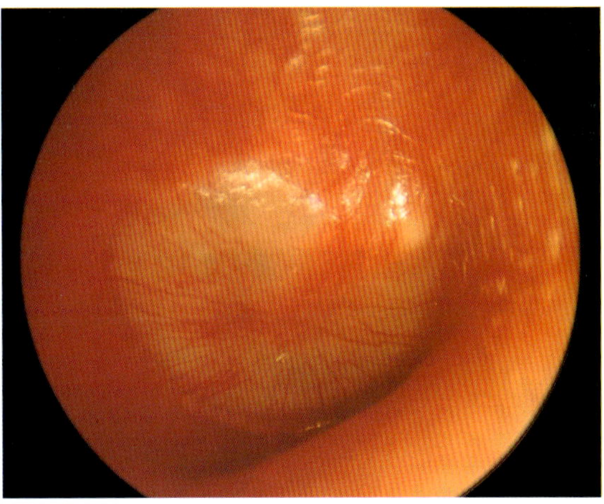

FIGURE 2.19 *Inflamed pars tensa due to right acute otitis media. External auditory canal is also inflamed.*

Q **Are the pars tensa and flaccida normal in consistency and colour?**

Figure 2.18 is an example where the tympanic membrane is intact and in a normal position but scarred. The diagnosis here is **healed otitis media**.

Figure 2.19 is an example where the tympanic membrane is intact and in a normal position but inflamed. The diagnosis here is **acute otitis media**.

Figure 2.20 is an example where the pars tensa is intact and in a relatively normal position but abnormal in colour, i.e. yellow. In this instance, this is because the middle ear is full of fluid: **otitis media with effusion**.

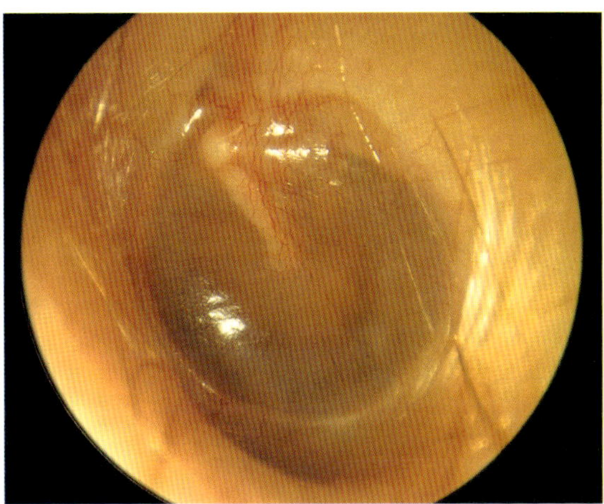

FIGURE 2.20 *Yellowish tympanic membrane due to left otitis media with effusion.*

MORE COMMON OTOSCOPIC DIAGNOSES

The inexperienced otoscopist is required to know the more common diagnoses and their usual otoscopic appearance. The latter can be extremely varied and multiple examples are illustrated in the symptom-based chapters. This chapter gives descriptions of the more common diagnoses alongside photographs of the classic otoscopic findings so that a basic understanding of the pathophysiology is available for reference when reading subsequent chapters.

CONDITIONS OF THE EXTERNAL EAR

OTITIS EXTERNA

Otitis externa is dermatitis of the external auditory canal which sometimes involves the pinna. In most this is an acute condition, often provoked by self-inflicted trauma in attempts to clean the ear out. Usually there is secondary colonisation of the inflamed skin by bacteria. In the more chronic condition, irritation or allergy, for example to topical medications, has to be considered.

The ear is uncomfortable and itchy making the patient want to scratch it or clean it out. In severe cases manipulation of the pinna causes discomfort and insertion of a speculum into the external auditory canal can be painful. There is usually a watery discharge and the canal skin is inflamed, oedematous and weepy

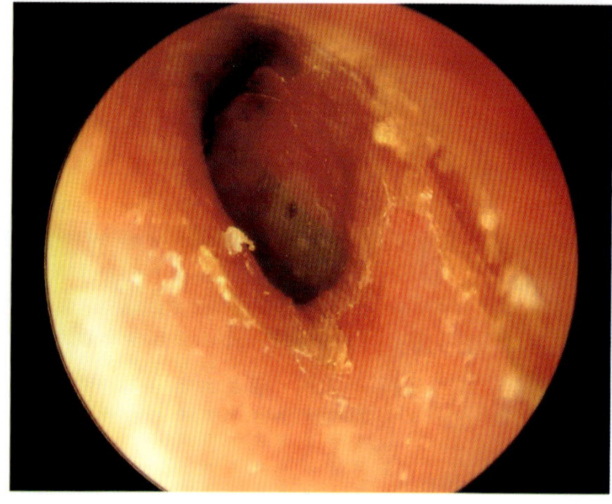

FIGURE 3.1 *Otitis externa (left) showing inflamed, oedematous and weepy canal skin.*

(Figure 3.1). Management is described in Chapter 6.

MIDDLE EAR CONDITIONS WITH ABNORMAL OTOSCOPY

ACUTE OTITIS MEDIA

Acute otitis media (AOM) is an acute inflammation of the mucosa of the middle ear and Eustachian tube which is common in infancy. The typical history is of a child, aged one to

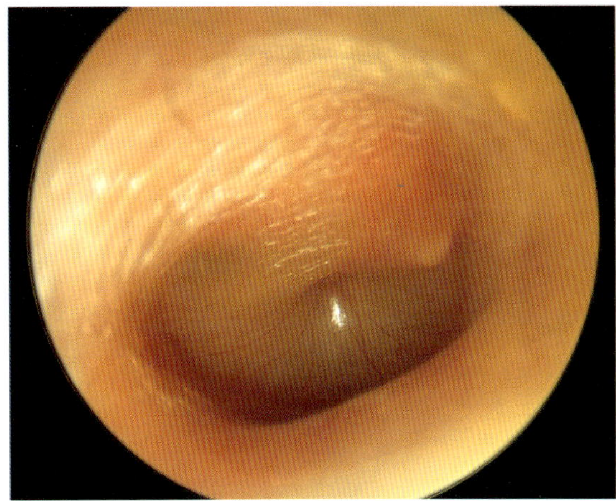

FIGURE 3.2 *Acute otitis media (right) showing generally inflamed and bulging pars tensa.*

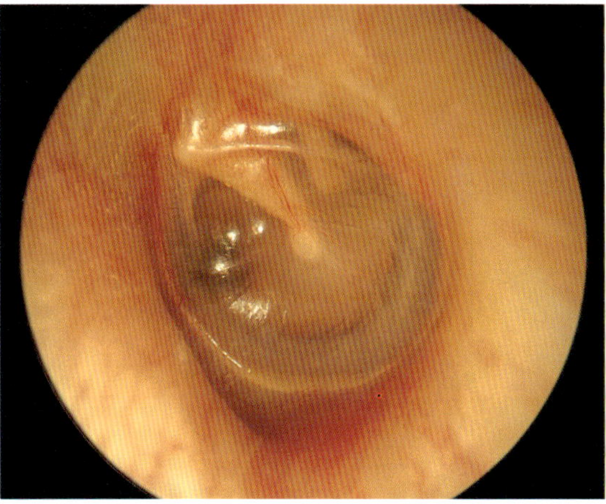

FIGURE 3.3 *Otitis media with effusion (right). In this ear this is evidenced by a more horizontal position of the handle of the malleus and a dull opaque pars tensa.*

three years, with a viral upper respiratory tract infection who wakes at night crying with a painful ear. It arises because the infection causes oedema and damage to the cilia of the respiratory epithelium of the Eustachian tube diminishing drainage of mucus from the middle ear. Secondary bacterial colonisation of the retained mucus may occur with the creation of what is in effect a middle ear abscess.

In the early stage, the tympanic membrane is intact but inflamed with prominent blood vessels on the handle of the malleus and the drum periphery. With the development of pus, the pars tensa becomes generally inflamed and begins to bulge (Figure 3.2). Natural resolution usually occurs by drainage of pus down the Eustachian tube or less frequently by perforating the tympanic membrane. Such perforations almost invariably heal spontaneously. Management is described in Chapter 6.

OTITIS MEDIA WITH EFFUSION

Otitis media with effusion (OME) is primarily a childhood condition where the middle ear is filled with a viscous fluid which impedes sound transmission through the middle ear. Various other terms have been used for this condition, such as secretory/serous otitis media, non-purulent chronic otitis media and glue ear.

The aetiology is multifactorial, including upper respiratory tract infections, previous acute otitis media, poor Eustachian tube function and adenoid hypertrophy.

The classical history is of a child, two to six years of age, who previously had normal hearing becoming dull of hearing. This may not be noticed by the parents and is often detected by childhood population screening. Occasionally there is otalgia. The natural history is one of episodes of resolution and recurrence followed by permanent resolution.

Otoscopically the tympanic membrane is intact but abnormal in position or colour. Unfortunately, these changes can be subtle and often difficult to detect. The negative middle ear pressure and the surface tension of the middle ear fluid tend to retract the drum into the middle ear cleft. This may often be evidenced by a more horizontal position of the handle of the malleus (Figure 3.3). The middle ear fluid itself causes a loss of translucency of the pars tensa which becomes dull and opaque. Pneumatic otoscopy reveals an immobile drum and tympanometry may be helpful in the diagnosis (see page 30). Management is discussed in Chapter 5.

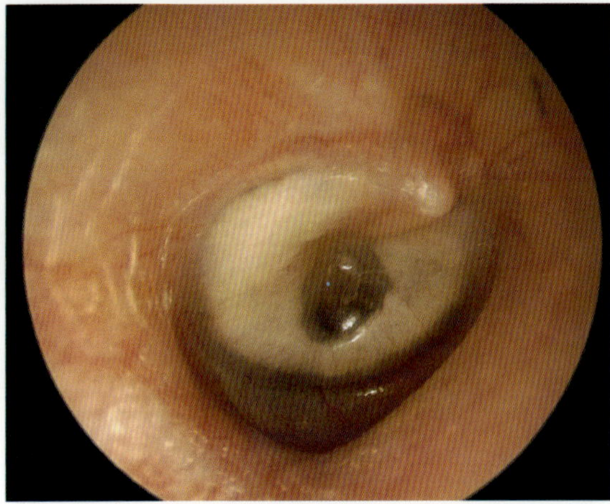

FIGURE 3.4 *Healed otitis media (right). In this ear there is a plaque of tympanosclerosis, mainly anterior but continuous inferiorly.*

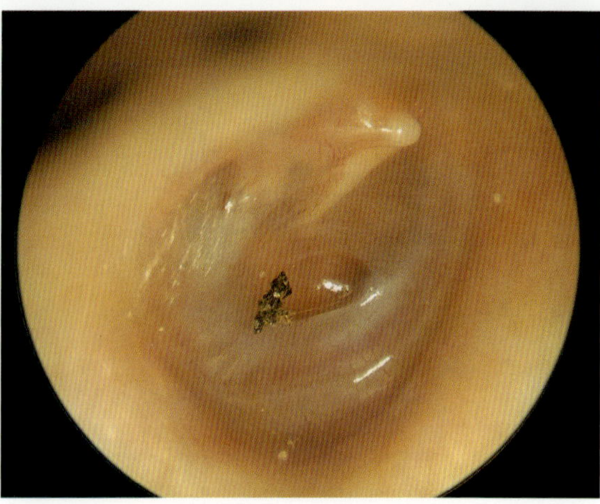

FIGURE 3.5 *Healed otitis media (right). In this ear there is a thin replacement membrane over what is presumed to be an old inferior perforation.*

HEALED OTITIS MEDIA

Healed otitis media (HOM) is where the pars tensa is intact but damaged. The pathology is tympanosclerosis when a white area affects a variable extent of the pars tensa and is due to hyaline degeneration of the fibrous collagen layer of the tympanic membrane together with secondary calcification. It can pass through various stages, from diffuse 'chalk' patches to well delineated plaques (Figure 3.4). Although not otoscopically evident when the tympanic membrane is intact, tympanosclerosis can also involve the ossicles.

The second main abnormality is that of replacement membranes (Figure 3.5) which are most easily thought of as perforations that have healed but with loss of the fibrous layer. This makes them particularly transparent.

HOM is the end result of previous middle ear conditions. The potential causes are many but include acute otitis media, otitis media with effusion, ventilating tubes (grommets) and other forms of tympanic membrane surgery. HOM is most commonly a chance finding on otoscopy. If there are any symptoms at all, it will be a hearing impairment of a conductive type. Whether surgery will alleviate this requires specialist appraisal (see pages 24–25). The alter-

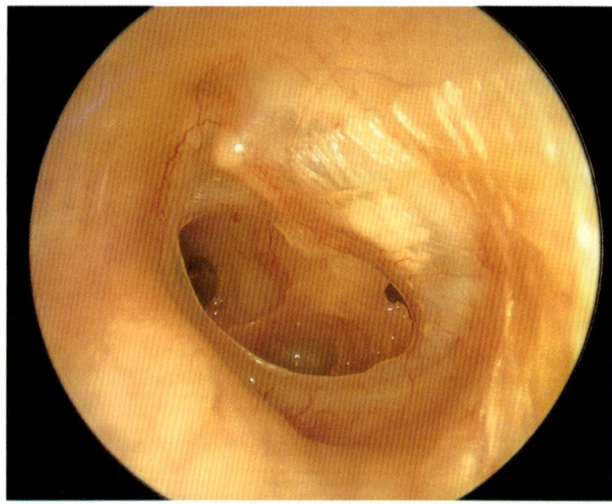

FIGURE 3.6 *Inactive left chronic otitis media. There is an anterior inferior pars tensa defect through which the middle ear mucosa can be seen to be normal, i.e. not inflamed.*

native is a hearing aid, which in ears with this diagnosis can be of considerable benefit.

CHRONIC OTITIS MEDIA

Chronic (suppurative) otitis media (COM) is due to chronic inflammation of the middle ear and mastoid which is associated with a permanent perforation (Figure 3.6) or retraction of

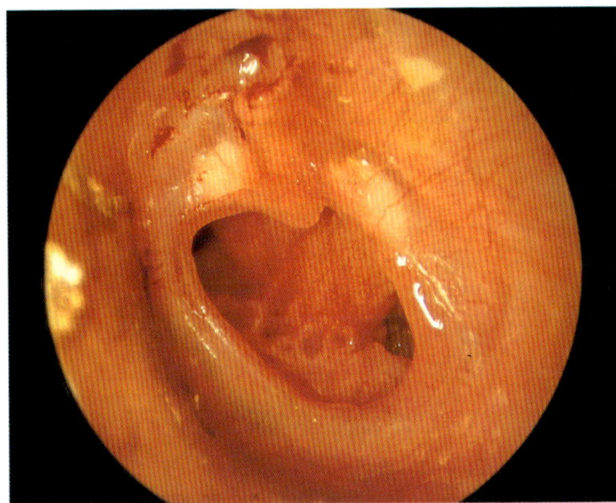

FIGURE 3.7 *Active left (mucosal) chronic otitis media. This photograph is taken after removal of mucopus and debris. There is a tympanic membrane defect through which the middle ear mucosa is seen to be inflamed and oedematous.*

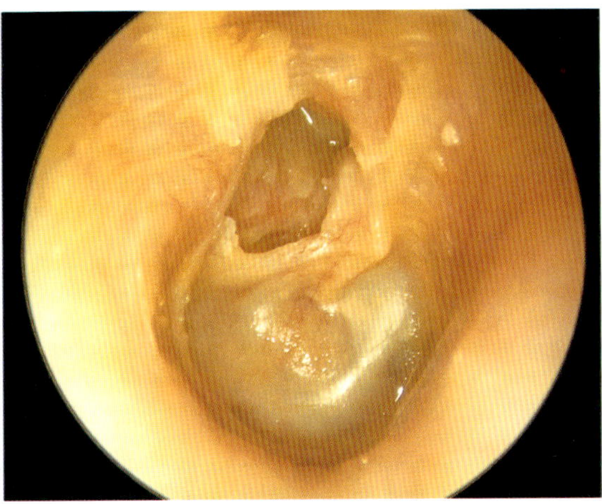

FIGURE 3.8 *Active right (squamous) chronic otitis media. The activity is centred in the attic in the pars flaccida rather than the pars tensa.*

the tympanic membrane. At any point in time, the ear may be active or inactive. This is the most important distinction to make in ears with COM because the management is different. In particular, ears that remain active should have a specialist assessment. This is because complications are not infrequent in ears that remain active. Specialist assessment can be difficult, in deciding both what anatomical areas are involved, and what the underlying pathology is. How much a non-specialist requires to know of these dilemmas is debatable but at least they ought to understand the pathological terminology and be able to examine the ear to ensure that they do not miss pathology.

When an ear is active, there is a foul smelling mucopurulent discharge which most commonly originates from an inflamed mucosa. The patient may or may not notice the discharge. Once the mucopus has been cleared, the otoscopist should be able to identify from which anatomical area of the ear it originated, namely the middle ear or the attic (or mastoid cavity if one has been surgically created).

When the middle ear is the site, the pars tensa will have a permanent defect, through which the inflamed middle ear mucosa should be seen (Figure 3.7). Such ears are more accurately defined as active (mucosal) COM. When the attic is the site, there is almost invariably some bone erosion of the attic wall and the mucopus originates from a retraction pocket of squamous epithelium surrounded by an inflamed mucosa (Figure 3.8). The retraction pocket is most easily thought of as an indrawn pars flaccida, and is usually filled with squamous epithelial debris. Such ears are more accurately described as active (squamous) COM or a cholesteatoma.

Management of active COM is described in Chapter 7.

There are also ears that when initially seen are inactive. These may or may not at some stage become active. Inactive COM, like active COM, can affect the middle ear or the attic but the former is more frequent. Thus in most inactive ears there is usually a permanent defect of the pars tensa but the middle ear mucosa seen through this is not inflamed and there is no mucopus (Figure 3.9). The presenting symptom is likely to be hearing impairment because of the less efficient middle ear sound conduction system. A hearing impairment is also likely in active ears but management of this

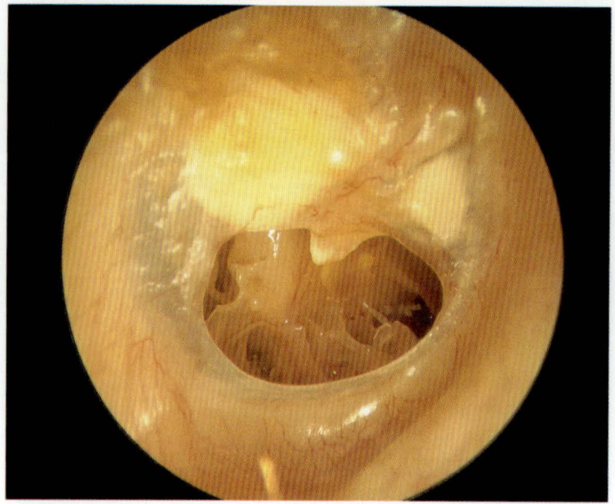

FIGURE 3.9 *Inactive right chronic otitis media. In this ear there is a permanent inferior defect of the pars tensa, through which the middle ear mucosa appears normal and not inflamed.*

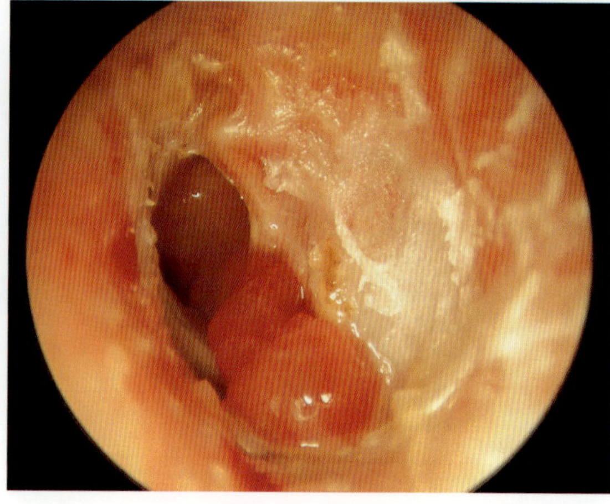

FIGURE 3.10 *Active left mucosal chronic otitis media. In this ear, in addition to the anterior pars tensa defect, the middle ear mucosa has hypertrophied to form protruding polyps.*

takes second place to that of the activity. The management of inactive COM is discussed in Chapter 4.

CHRONIC OTITIS MEDIA – SPECIALIST

In adults chronic otitis media is a common otoscopic diagnosis having an incidence of 5% in the British population (Browning and Gatehouse, 1992). Otoscopically there are many different appearances, but thorough toilet and examination with a microscope normally make interpretation less difficult. Different terms have been used to describe ears with chronic (suppurative) otitis media; Table 3.1 summarises the ones most frequently used (Browning, 1995). The first distinction to be made is whether the ear is currently active and, if so, what the pathological process is. There are

two main variants of active, and two of inactive, disease.

Active mucosal chronic otitis media

Here the middle ear mucosa is inflamed to a variable degree, sometimes with the development of granulation tissue and polyps (Figure 3.10). The mucosa around the ossicular chain is sometimes particularly affected. The pars tensa is perforated to a variable extent and the ossicular chain may or may not be eroded (Figures 3.11 and 3.12). The classical but now mainly discarded term for such ears was tubotympanic disease. These were considered 'safe'.

Active squamous chronic otitis media – cholesteatoma

The inflammatory process in such ears is most commonly of the pars flaccida in the attic and

TABLE 3.1 *Classification of types of chronic (suppurative) otitis media (COM)*

	Pathological	Clinical	Traditional
Active	Mucosal COM	Active COM	Tubotympanic, 'safe'
	Squamous COM	Cholesteatoma	Attico-antral, 'unsafe'
Inactive	Mucosal COM	Inactive COM	
	Squamous COM	Retraction pocket	

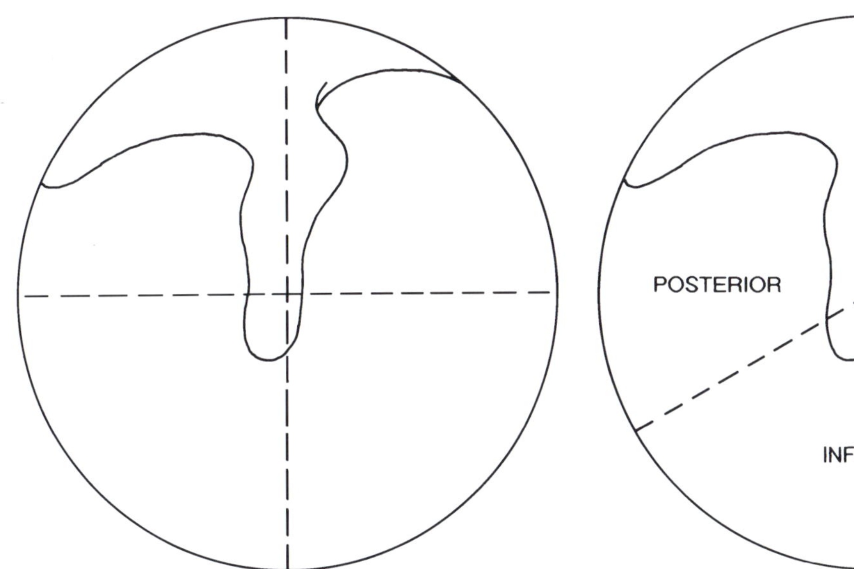

FIGURE 4.2 *Drawing of the four quadrants of pars tensa. Right ear.*

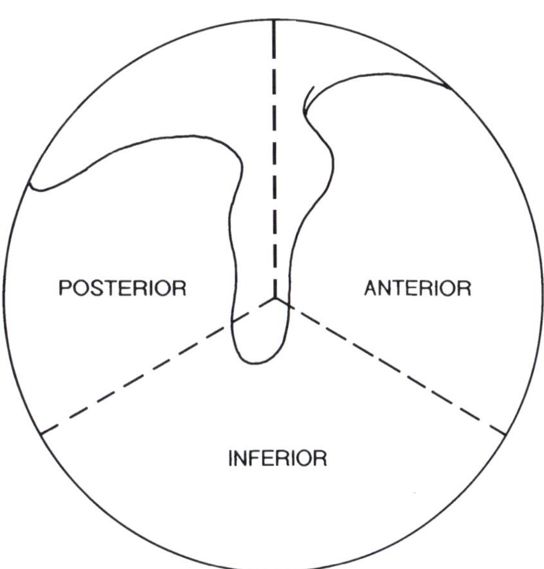

FIGURE 4.3 *Drawing of the three thirds of pars tensa. Right ear.*

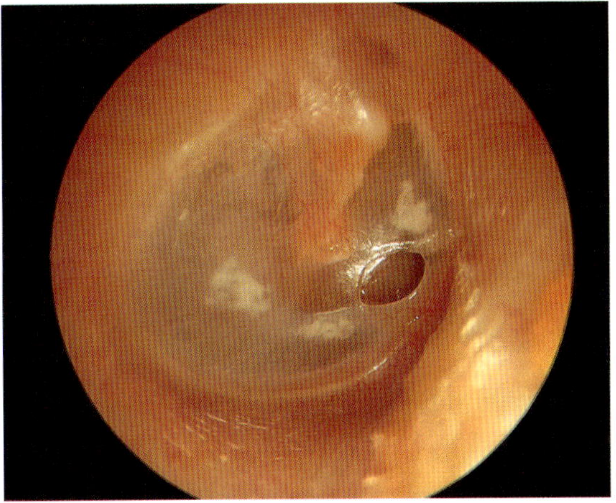

FIGURE 4.4 *Anterior perforation in inactive (mucosal) chronic otitis media. Right ear.*

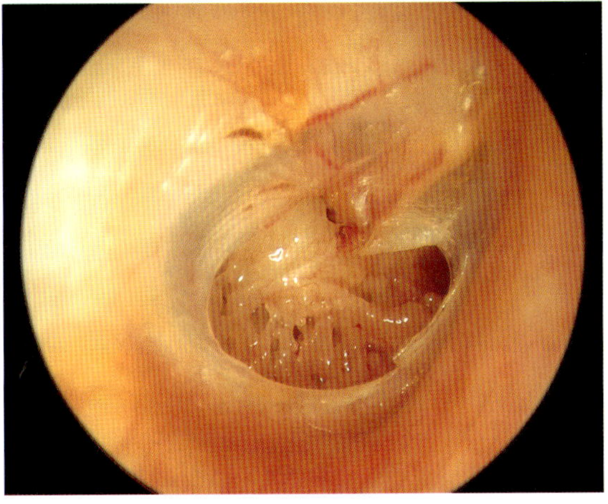

FIGURE 4.5 *Inferior perforation in inactive (mucosal) chronic otitis media. Right ear.*

disease affected the pars flaccida. Unfortunately others have subsequently used central and marginal perforations in a different context, using it to describe whether a defect of the pars tensa extends to the annulus or not. Some consider the annulus has to be absent to make a perforation marginal. Otoscopically this sometimes might appear to be the case but it is rare to find the annulus absent at surgery. Thus, for example, in an anterior perforation, it may appear to extend to the bony margin (Figure 4.11) but

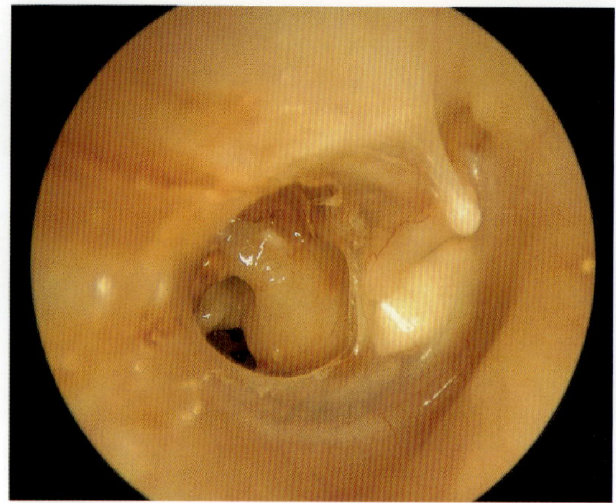

FIGURE 4.6 *Posterior perforation in inactive (mucosal) chronic otitis media. Right ear.*

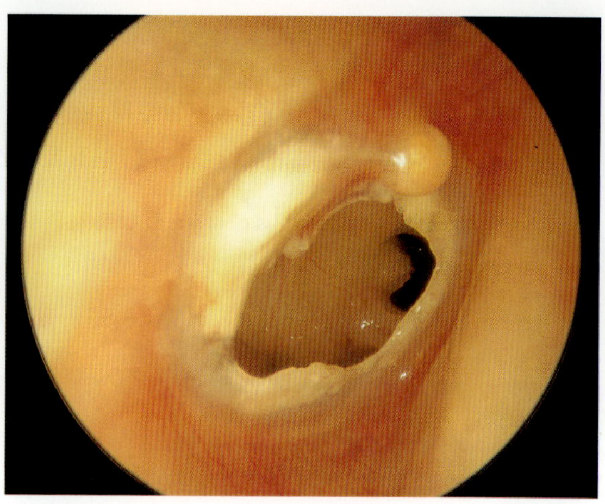

FIGURE 4.7 *Antero-inferior perforation in inactive (mucosal) chronic otitis media. Right ear.*

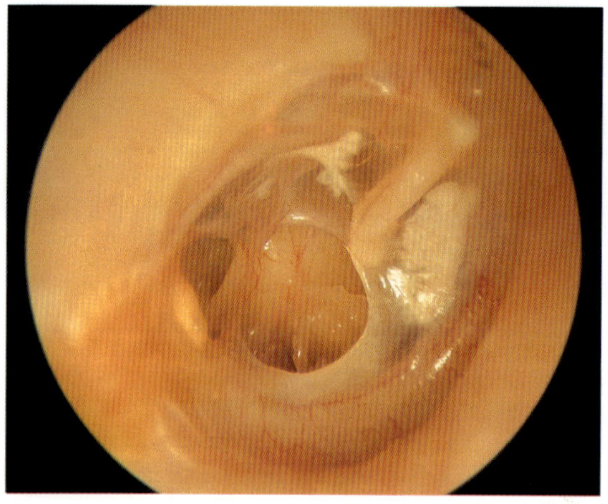

FIGURE 4.8 *Postero-inferior perforation in inactive (mucosal) chronic otitis media. Right ear.*

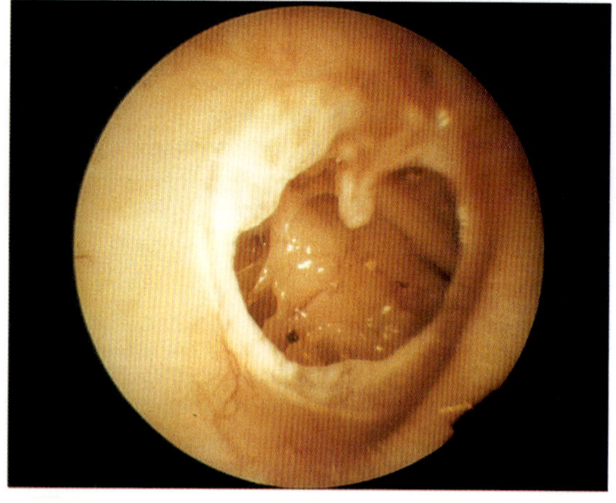

FIGURE 4.9 *Subtotal perforation in inactive (mucosal) chronic otitis media. Right ear.*

when adequate surgical exposure is achieved, this is found not to be the case (Figure 4.12).

Size of defect

In addition to stating where the perforation is, it is usual to say what percentage of the tympanic membrane is affected. Thus Figure 4.4 is a 10% anterior, Figure 4.5 is a 60% inferior, Figure 4.6 a 40% posterior perforation and Figure 4.9 a 95% (total) perforation.

Ossicular chain

In chronic otitis media the most common ossicular chain abnormality is erosion of the long process of the incus. In posterior perforations it is frequently possible to see the incudostapedial joint and to state whether erosion has occurred. Figure 4.13 is an example where it is eroded. Figure 4.14 an example where it is partially eroded and Figure 4.15 an example where it is not. Sometimes the stapes superstructure is also

CENTRAL PERFORATIONS

MARGINAL RETRACTIONS (Perforations)

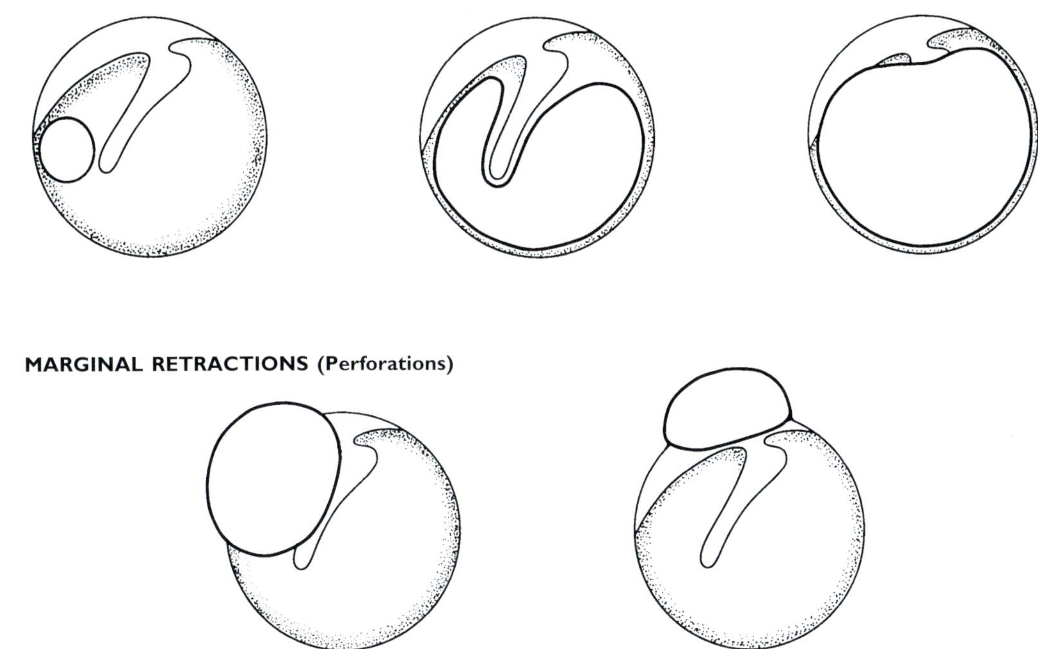

FIGURE 4.10 *Drawing, after Diamant (1982), to show classic distinction between marginal and central perforations. Right ear.*

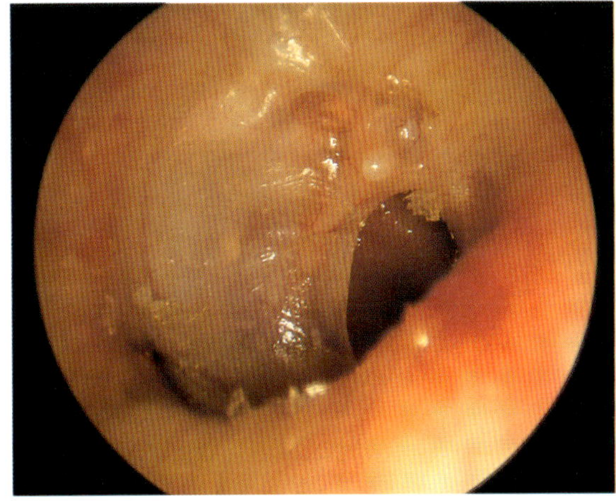

FIGURE 4.11 *Anterior perforation with absent annulus. Slightly inflamed. Right ear.*

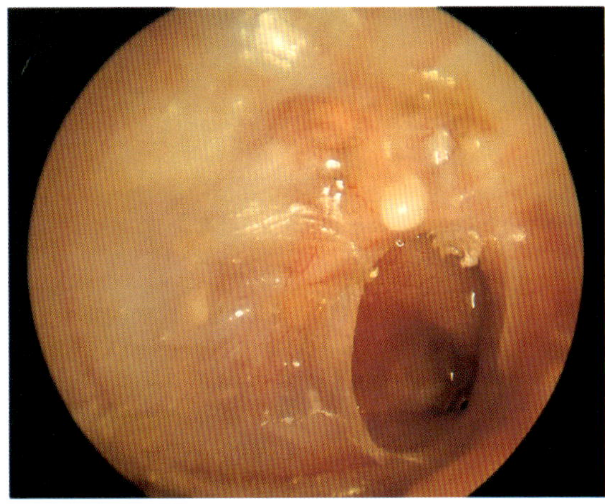

FIGURE 4.12 *Same ear as Figure 4.11 but better view anteriorly.*

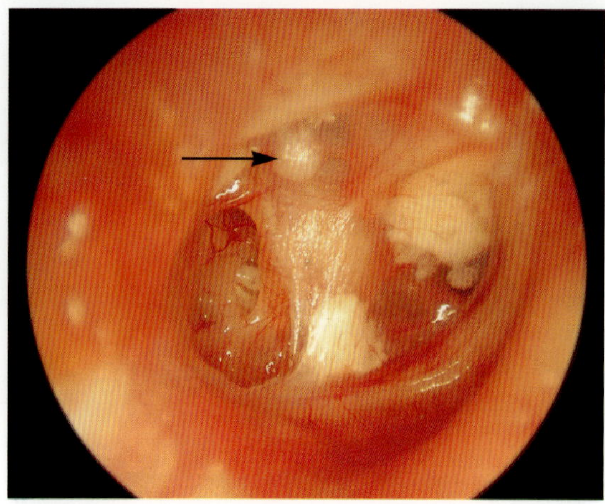

FIGURE 4.13 *Eroded long process of incus in inactive (mucosal) chronic otitis media. The stapes remains with the tympanic membrane retracted onto it (arrowed). Right ear.*

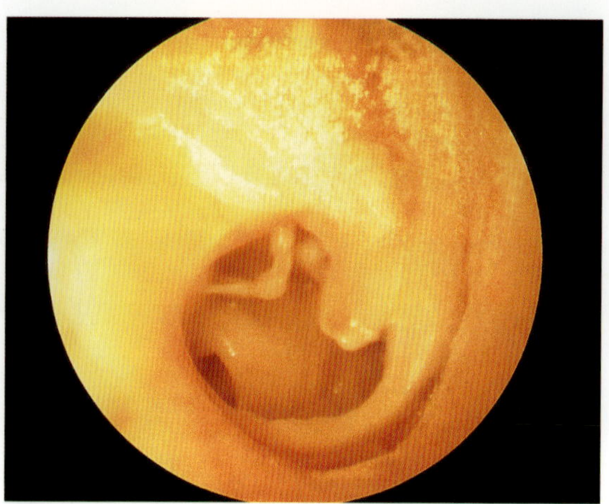

FIGURE 4.14 *Partially eroded long process of incus in inactive (mucosal) chronic otitis media. Right ear.*

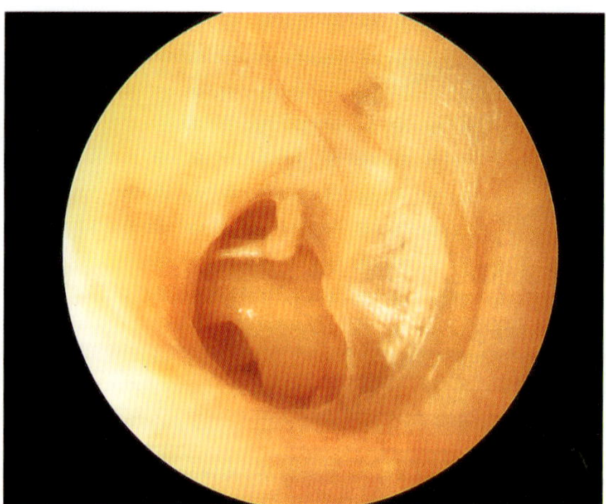

FIGURE 4.15 *Not eroded long process of incus in inactive (mucosal) chronic otitis media. Right ear.*

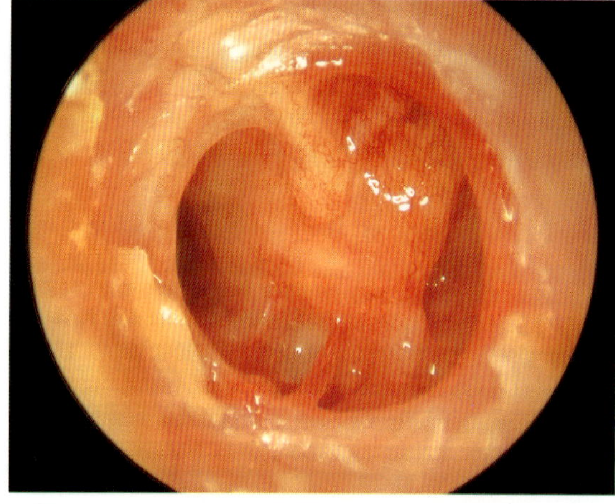

FIGURE 4.16 *Erosion stapes superstructure in inactive (mucosal) chronic otitis media. Right ear.*

eroded (Figure 4.16). In inferior and total perforations the handle of the malleus may be eroded (Figure 4.17). Rather surprisingly this need not be associated with erosion of the long process of the incus.

The appearance of any remaining pars tensa should be noted because if tympanosclerotic (see Figures 4.6 and 4.7), the ossicular chain may also be fixed by tympanosclerosis. Most frequently this occurs around the head of the malleus and body of incus but it can also fix the stapes in the oval window

Look at branch 4.1A

If the tympanic membrane is intact, it should be decided ⑤ whether it is retracted and abnormal

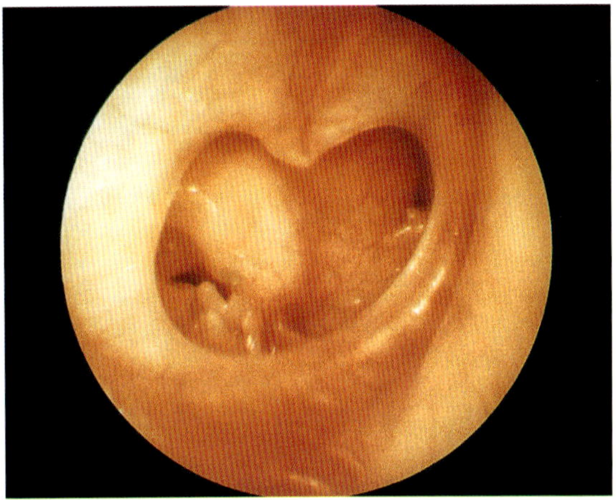

FIGURE 4.17 *Erosion handle of malleus in inactive (mucosal) chronic otitis media. Right ear.*

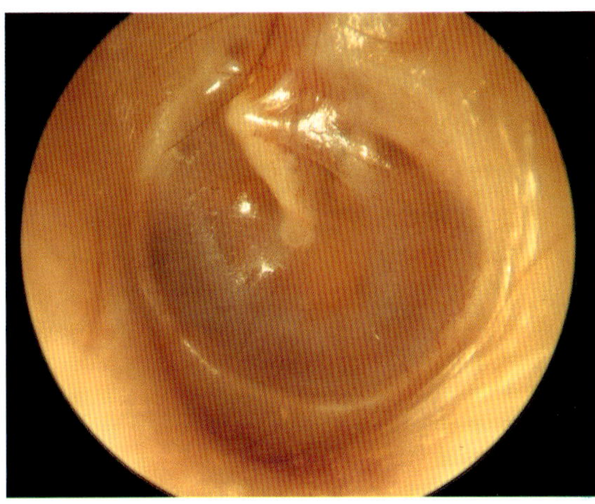

FIGURE 4.18 *Retracted, yellow pars flaccida in otitis media with effusion. Left ear.*

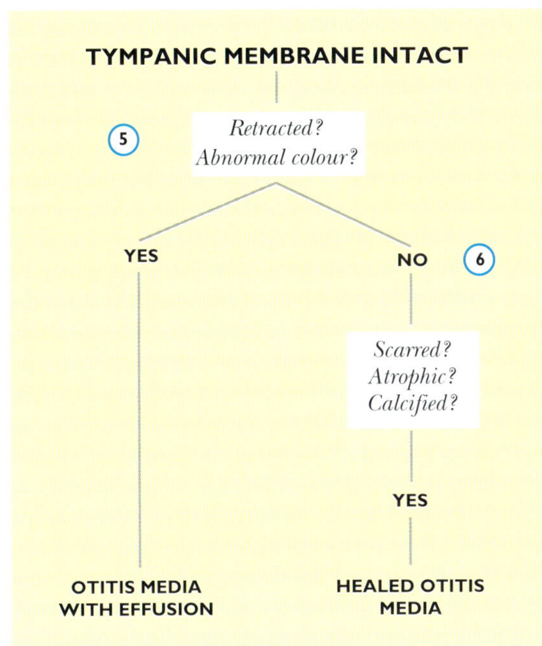

Branch 4.1A

in colour. Otitis media with effusion is the diagnosis if the pars tensa is generally retracted and slightly yellow in colour (Figure 4.18).

OTITIS MEDIA WITH EFFUSION

Otitis media is less common in adults than in children (see Chapter 5). It sometimes occurs temporarily following an upper respiratory tract infection but sometimes it is chronic. In most of the latter the aetiology is uncertain. However, chronic nasal disease and post-nasal space tumours have to be excluded before ascribing it an idiopathic diagnosis. Hence, referral to a specialist is mandatory in chronic cases. The otoscopic findings in adults are as variable as they are in children (see page 30).

Otitis media with effusion – specialist

After a full clinical examination, including endoscopy to exclude nasal or post-nasal pathology, the specialist has to decide on management. The severity of the hearing impairment will be assessed by pure-tone audiometry and if the reported disability merits management either a long-term ventilating tube (grommet) (Figure 4.19) is inserted or a hearing aid provided. There are many different varieties of long-term grommets, the most common having large flanges which help to prevent extrusion. The reason that long-term grommets are used in adults with OME is that

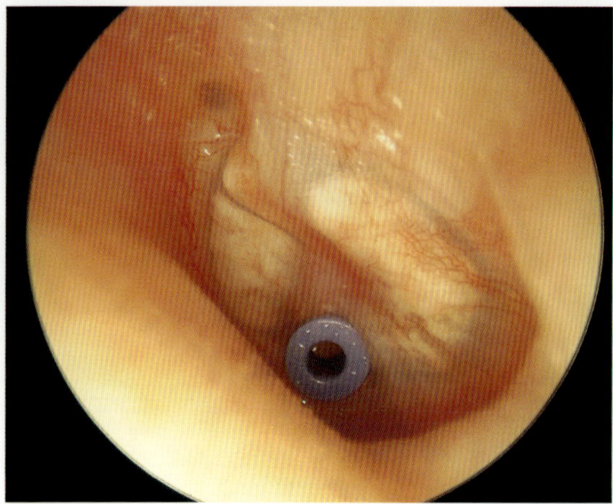

FIGURE 4.19 *Long-term ventilating tube (umbra minor). Pars tensa and flaccida now in normal position. Gross tympanosclerosis. Left ear.*

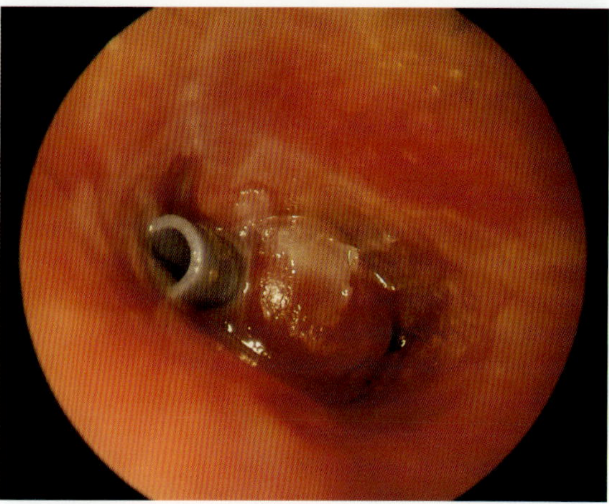

FIGURE 4.20 *Secondary infection around long-term ventilating tube. Left ear.*

in them the condition tends to be protracted over several years rather than months as it is in children. As with grommets of any type, secondary infection is not uncommon (Figure 4.20) but this frequently settles with aural toilet and the use of topical steroid and antibiotic ear drops.

> *Look at branch 4.1A*

If an intact tympanic membrane is abnormal but not retracted it will be because of its consistency ⑥. It might be scarred, atrophic or calcified, all of which can be present in healed otitis media.

HEALED OTITIS MEDIA

In HOM there is evidence of previous episodes of otitis media. The pars tensa is abnormal, perhaps having areas of tympanosclerosis and of atrophy (Figure 4.21). As there is no likelihood of such ears progressing to active COM, the management is solely of any associated conductive hearing impairment.

Healed otitis media – specialist

In HOM the main decision a specialist has to make is whether middle ear surgery is likely to alleviate any hearing disability. Tympanosclerosis and healed perforations by themselves are unlikely to cause a material conductive

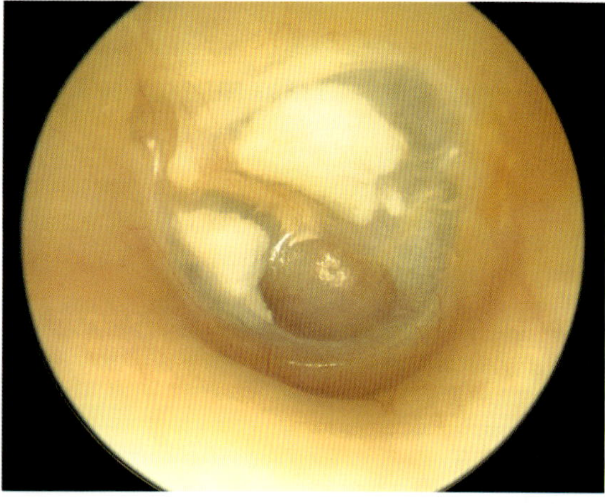

FIGURE 4.21 *Tympanosclerotic tympanic membrane in healed otitis media. Left ear.*

impairment. This is because the area of the tympanic membrane that collects sound vibrations and transmits them to the handle of the malleus is not reduced. Hence the piston sound conduction system of the middle ear, which utilises an area difference between the tympanic membrane and the oval window, is not greatly affected. If the air–bone gap is greater than

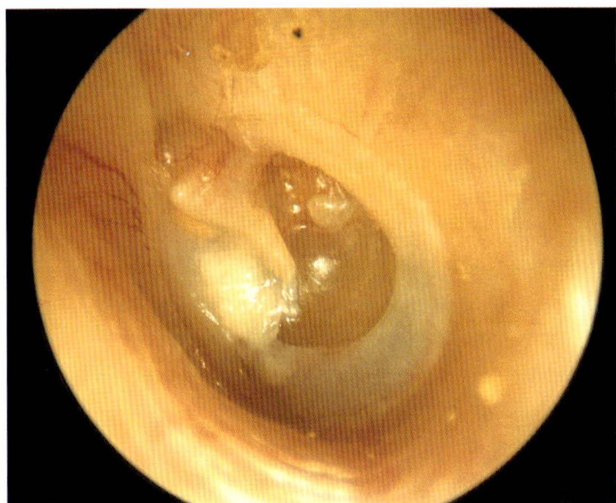

FIGURE 4.22 *Erosion of long process of incus seen through atrophic membrane in healed otitis media. Left ear.*

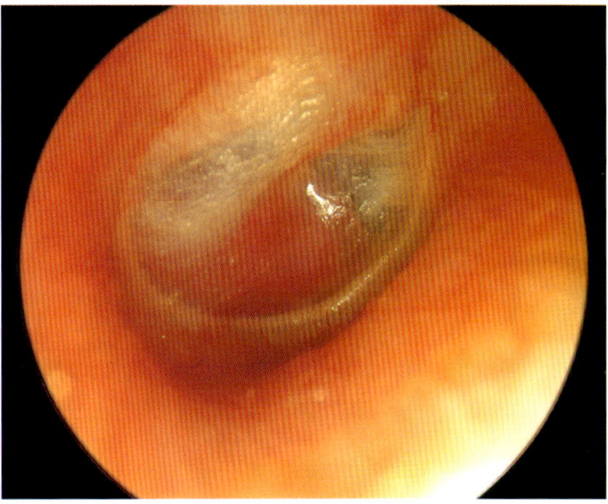

FIGURE 4.23 *Glomus tympanicum (right). Red, pulsatile flush of inferior pars tensa. 'Rising sun' appearance.*

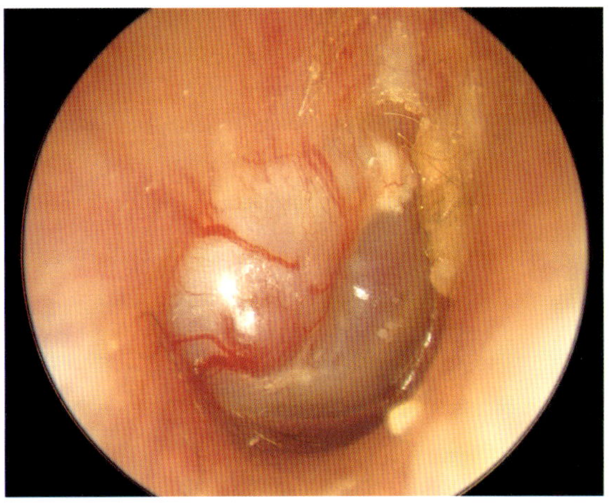

FIGURE 4.24 *Glomus jugulare (right). Red pulsatile swelling of posterior pars tensa. Radiology confirms involvement of jugular foramen.*

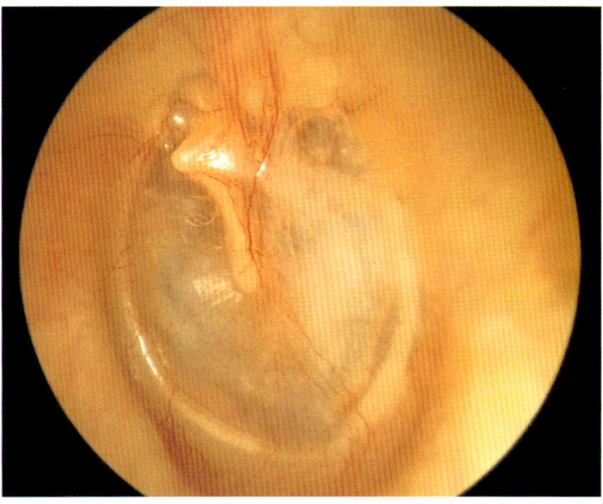

FIGURE 4.25 *Left stapedotomy. Posterosuperior canal wall was curretted.*

10 dB, ossicular chain problems become more likely. This can be because of tympanosclerotic fixation of an intact chain, which is not usually considered surgically correctable. The alternative is that the ossicular chain is disrupted. This is eminently correctable by surgery. The distinction between these two types of problem can only be made on exploratory tympanotomy unless the ossicular chain can be seen through the tympanic membrane (Figure 4.22).

SPECIALIST – CONSIDER ALTERNATIVE DIAGNOSIS

GLOMUS TUMOURS

These are relatively uncommon middle ear vascular tumours that present most frequently with a hearing impairment and pulsatile tinnitus. The size of the tumour varies from being confined to the middle ear (glomus tympanicum) to surrounding the jugular bulb (glomus jugulare) when it can be associated with lower cranial nerve palsies due to bone erosion. The distinction is made by radiology. In both, the tympanic membrane is red and pulsates (Figures 4.23 and 4.24). Larger tumours cause the tympanic membrane to bulge and they may extend into the canal. Management is tailored to the individual patient, varying from observation, to local or radical surgery, and radiotherapy.

SUMMARY FOR NON-SPECIALISTS WHEN OTOSCOPY IS ABNORMAL

If an otoscopic abnormality is detected in an individual being examined because of a hearing impairment, referral to a specialist is advisable, the exception being when otitis media with effusion is a temporary sequela of an upper respiratory tract infection. Clinical tests of hearing (see page 87) help to confirm that an impairment is present and whether it is unilateral or bilateral. They are not particularly helpful in deciding whether to refer, because the main criteria are the degree of disability the patient reports and their willingness to be referred. Tuning fork tests are rarely carried out by non-specialists.

SUMMARY FOR SPECIALISTS WHEN OTOSCOPY IS ABNORMAL

A pure-tone audiogram is essential to help decide management. The magnitude of the air–bone gap, taken in conjunction with the otoscopic appearance, will decide whether surgery has a role. It is generally held that an air–bone gap of 10 dB or more over 0.5, 1 and 2 kHz has to be present for surgery to be considered. In COM the type of surgery required can often be determined by otoscopy in conjunction with the magnitude of the air–bone gap. Figures 4.4 and 4.5 are examples where a myringoplasty is all that would be necessary if the air–bone gap was 15 dB. On the other hand, Figure 4.6 is an example where an ossiculoplasty is likely to be necessary if the air–bone gap was 35 dB. This is because a gap of this size suggests a high possibility of erosion of the long process of the incus. In Figure 4.7 tympanosclerotic fixation of the ossicular chain is a possibility to consider if the air–bone gap was 35 dB.

Having decided what surgery might be required and assuming that the surgical skills are available and proven, the next question is what is likely to be achieved in terms of reducing the patient's disability (Browning *et al.*, 1991). This is a complex issue but mainly depends on two factors. The first is whether the ear to be operated on has a mixed or a pure conductive impairment. If the former, a hearing aid will still be desirable, even if surgery is technically successful. The second factor is the degree of symmetry of hearing. When this is symmetrical any improvement in the air conduction thresholds in one ear will be noticed and be of benefit to the patient. When the thresholds are asymmetrical, the poorer hearing ear will be the one operated upon and though the degree of closure of the air–bone gap may be similar, the benefit will be less. This is because, in most circumstances, the better hearing ear (i.e. the non-operated ear) is the main determinant of disability. So unless the operated ear becomes the better hearing ear, the non-operated ear will remain the main hearing ear. Thus, surgery on a unilateral conductive impairment will not be so noticeably of benefit to the patient as would surgery on a bilateral symmetrical impairment.

Look at branch 4.1B

WHEN OTOSCOPY IS NORMAL

Having found that both ears are otoscopically normal, the next step ⑦ is to assess informally the hearing by free-field voice testing (see page 87). This indicates the degree of impairment in each ear which, taken in conjunction with patient report, will decide whether the hearing is symmetrical. If yes, the hearing impairment is most likely to be sensorineural though a conductive impairment due to otosclerosis is a possibility. Most non-specialists would not try to distinguish the two by tuning-fork tests but would rely upon an otolaryngologist to make the diagnosis.

If the hearing is reported as or found to be asymmetrical then referral to a specialist is important. This is because an acoustic neuroma has to be excluded (see page 28).

In most countries there are two alternative routes to seeking a specialist opinion for a hearing impaired adult with normal otoscopy: the first is to an otolaryngologist. This is considered the route of choice in younger patients because in them there is a higher possibility of otosclerosis. It is also the preferred route for those with asymmetrical hearing. The alternative route is directly to a hearing aid dispenser, either commercial or, as in the United Kingdom, directly to a hospital audiology department. This route is appropriate for the more elderly who are most likely to have a sensorineural impairment for which a hearing aid is the sole management option.

SPECIALIST – LOOK AT BRANCH 4.1B

Having confirmed that the tympanic membranes are indeed normal, the specialist's initial task is to decide whether the impairment is conductive, sensorineural or mixed. This is best done by pure-tone audiometry with accurate masking, particularly of the bone conduction. Many would still carry out tuning fork tests, particularly the Rinne test (see page 88). If a material conductive component is identified the most likely diagnosis is otosclerosis, unless the impairment followed a severe head injury (see page 76).

OTOSCLEROSIS

Otosclerosis remains a presumptive diagnosis unless the ear is surgically explored as there is no consistent way, either audiological or radiological, of confirming the diagnosis. Having

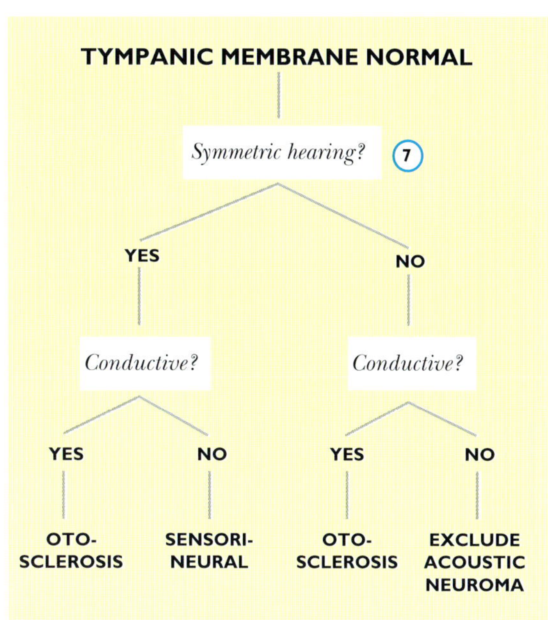

Branch 4.1B

made the diagnosis the specialist's decision is whether to recommend surgery, a hearing aid, or both. In experienced hands, especially if a small fenestra stapedotomy is performed with a microdrill or laser, the air–bone gap can be closed in the majority with a low incidence of temporary postoperative imbalance. The potential benefit to the patient in terms of lessening of disability and eliminating the need for a hearing aid is the same as discussed in patients with other middle ear conditions. Postoperatively the tympanic membrane is sometimes scarred and the posterosuperior canal partly removed (Figure 4.25). Occasionally the wire of the prosthesis can also be seen.

SYMMETRICAL SENSORINEURAL IMPAIRMENT

The patient's history should identify any factors that might be responsible for the impairment. Thus noise exposure should be inquired about, as should any illness which might have necessitated potentially ototoxic drugs, such as aminoglycosides, being administered. Ascertaining predisposing factors is of interest but not of management significance, unless they are still occurring, e.g. noise exposure. The management is with a hearing aid or aids and appropriate instruction in their use.

ASYMMETRICAL SENSORINEURAL IMPAIRMENT

Unless there is a definite aetiology such as a severe head injury with skull fracture, investigation to rule out an acoustic neuroma is mandatory. This is most reliably done by magnetic resonance imaging (MRI) of the temporal bone, though electric response audiometry or computed tomography (CT) scanning can be used instead.

CHAPTER 5

HEARING IMPAIRMENT IN CHILDREN

THE GENERAL DIAGNOSTIC PROBLEM

Hearing impairments in children can be sensorineural or conductive in type. Sensorineural impairments are almost invariably permanent. They can be unilateral or bilateral and of a severity ranging from mild to total. The majority of these are congenital in origin. Without amplification and appropriate rehabilitation, children with bilateral severe or total impairments will fail to develop normal speech and language – the classic prelingual deaf and dumb child. Hence early detection is important. There are many problems with early detection programmes. Neonatal screening is designed to detect such children before they leave hospital, the practical problem being that there is no cheap, sensitive and specific hearing test at this age. Techniques such as brain stem audiometry and evoked oto-acoustic emissions are time consuming and, though sensitive, lack specificity. This is because, as well as detecting the majority of infants with a severe sensorineural impairment, they also detect children with OME. This, in most instances, is transitory and should not cause concern. One way of reducing the screening workload and increasing the proportion of sensorineural impairments detected is to screen children particularly at risk of a congenital impairment. Such children are those with a family history of hearing impairment, mothers with prenatal infections such as rubella, those hypoxic at birth, those given aminoglycosides and those with other congenital abnormalities, e.g. Down's syndrome. However, confining screening to 'at risk' children identifies only 50% of congenitally deaf children.

Sensorineural impairments can also be acquired in early childhood from meningitis and viral infections such as mumps and measles, which are often subclinical. Hence, as well as neonatal screening, it is conventional in many countries for health visitors to carry out free-field 'distraction testing' in all children at about nine months of age. Unfortunately such testing is not simple (McCormack, 1988) and if poorly performed will miss severely impaired children. Another drawback in such testing frequently identifies children with transient OME. Perhaps the most important aspect to note is any concern that the parents or grandparents may express because the child does not appear to be as aware of environmental sounds as normal children, or is slow to develop speech.

Look at summary tree 5.1

Otoscopy in children is never particularly easy, but can be made more difficult if they become frightened. Getting the mother to hold the child's head against their chest with a firm hand can be helpful (Figure 5.1) Another problem is wax, which may partially or totally obstruct the view. Its removal by syringing very frequently disturbs the child.

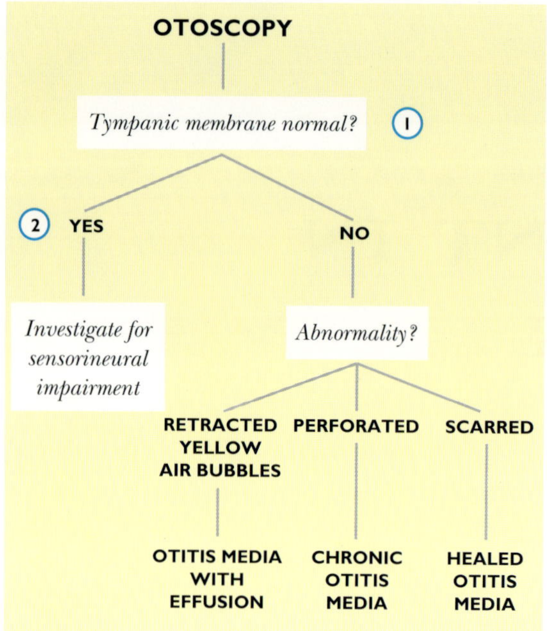

Summary tree 5.1 Hearing impairment in children.

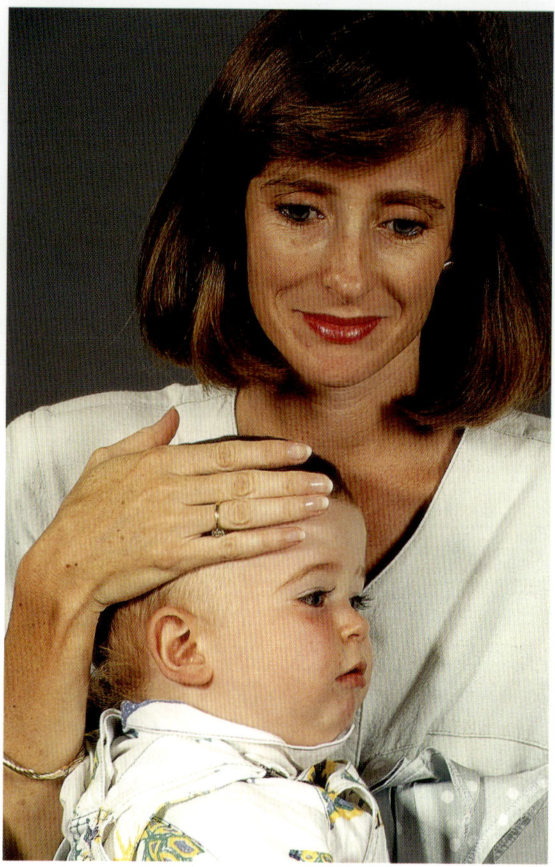

FIGURE 5.1 *Method of holding child's head still against chest.*

The two main diagnoses to consider in children with a hearing impairment are OME and a sensorineural impairment. The distinction is made on otoscopy by assessing the tympanic membrane ①. If this is normal ②, the child should be investigated for a sensorineural impairment. If abnormal ③, there are three main diagnoses to consider and the distinction rests on what the abnormality is, but the most likely diagnosis is OME. COM and HOM are diagnoses in older children. How to make these diagnoses is discussed in Chapter 4. The current chapter concentrates on OME and its potential sequelae.

HOW TO MAKE A DIAGNOSIS OF OTITIS MEDIA WITH EFFUSION

Unfortunately, the otoscopic appearances of otitis media with effusion can be extremely varied and, for the non-specialist who usually does not have access to pneumatic otoscopy and tympanometry, this can give rise to diagnostic problems. The easy answer is to refer children on to a specialist when in doubt, but this could create an unnecessarily large specialist workload because, by the time the child is seen, the otitis media will often have resolved spontaneously.

The following is a series of questions that should be asked when assessing the tympanic membrane to detect otitis media with effusion.

Q *Is the pars tensa retracted?*

This is most frequently evident by the handle of the malleus being in a more horizontal position than normal (Figures 5.2–5.5), rather than the membrane itself appearing more cone shaped. With progressive degrees of pars tensa retraction, a neoannular fold can develop (arrowed in Figure 5.5).

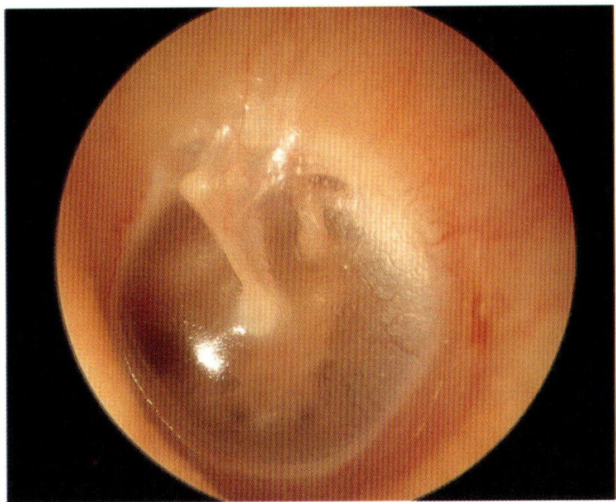

FIGURE 5.2 *Otitis media with effusion (left). Malleus handle in normal position.*

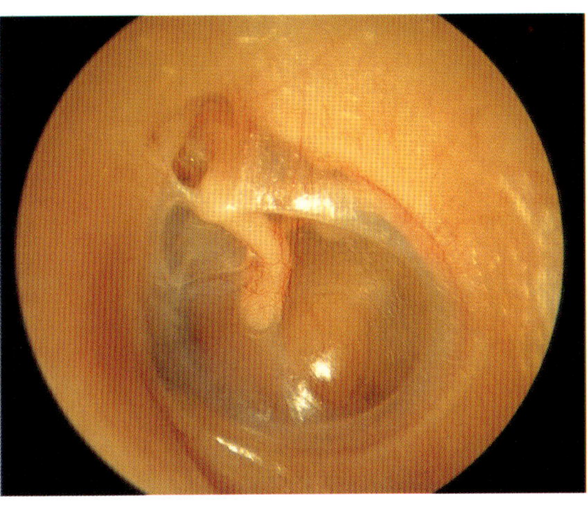

FIGURE 5.3 *Otitis media with effusion (left). Malleus handle slightly retracted.*

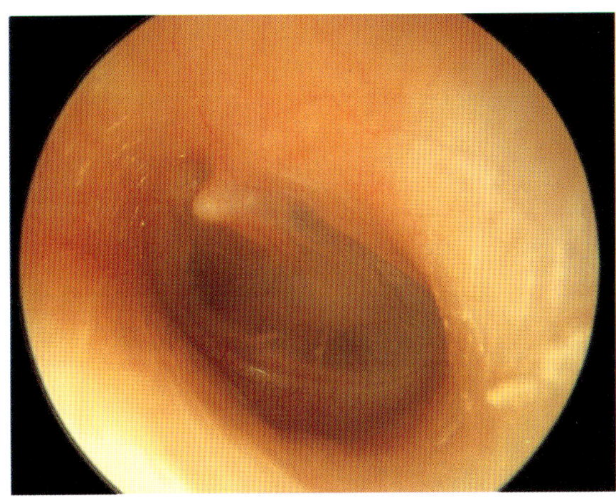

FIGURE 5.4 *Otitis media with effusion (left). Malleus handle markedly retracted.*

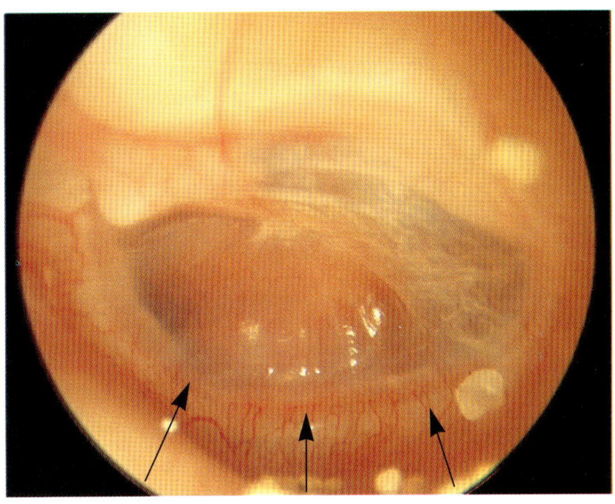

FIGURE 5.5 *Severely retracted position of malleus handle in otitis media with effusion. Left ear. As retraction develops a neoannular fold may develop (arrow).*

Q Is the colour normal?

Middle ear fluid can affect the colour in subtle ways ranging from yellowish (Figure 5.6), through clear (Figure 5.7) to bluish (Figure 5.8).

Q Is there a fluid level or air bubbles?

These findings are relatively uncommon (Figures 5.9 and 5.10).

In some ears there is a combination of all three findings.

Whether it is possible to informally test the hearing by free-field voice testing (see page 87) depends on the child's age and whether he will respond. Masking is not necessary because all one needs to know is whether the child is hearing-impaired in the better hearing ear. This

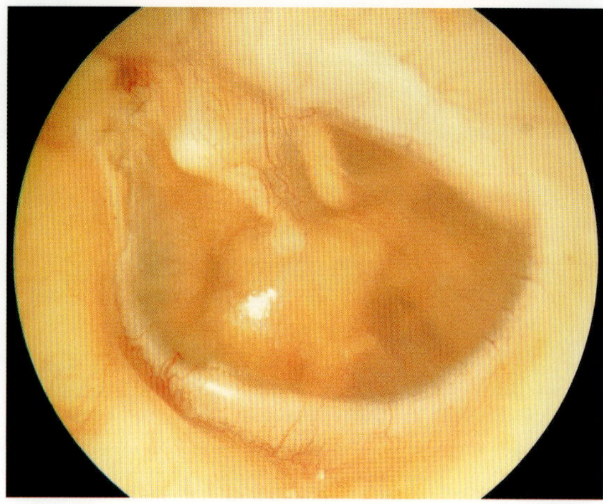

FIGURE 5.6 *Left tympanic membrane in otitis media with effusion showing yellowish colour.*

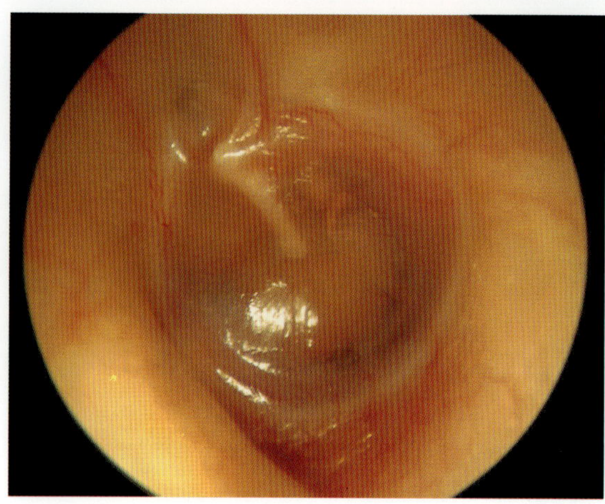

FIGURE 5.7 *Left tympanic membrane in otitis media with effusion showing clear colour.*

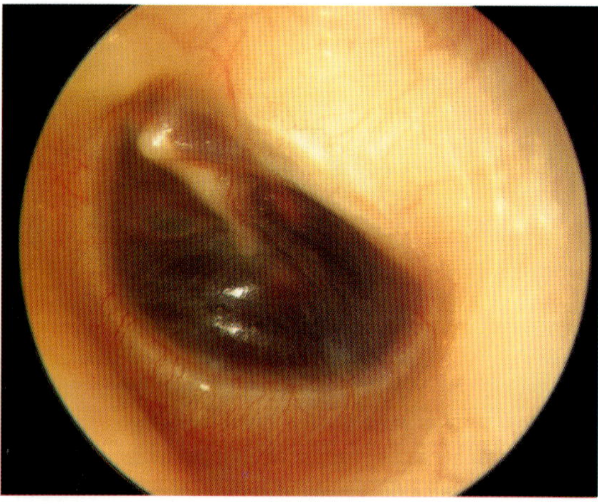

FIGURE 5.8 *Left tympanic membrane in otitis media with effusion showing bluish colour.*

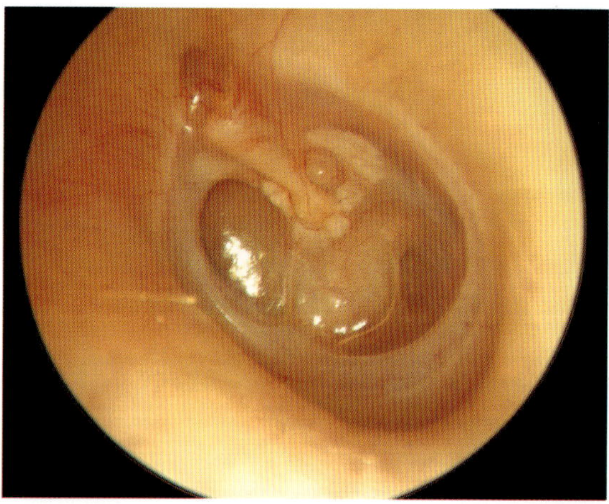

FIGURE 5.9 *Fluid level in otitis media with effusion. Left ear.*

is the case if they cannot hear a whispered voice at 60 cm (2 ft) when the tester is out of vision. The child can be engaged in conversation and asked a series of simple questions. These can require an answer, such as 'How old are you?' or just a response, such as 'Where is your nose?'. The questions can gradually be posed in a whisper from behind the child, 60 cm from the back of their head. If the child responds in this position, there is no serious concern regarding a hearing impairment causing speech and language delay.

At this stage there will often be considerable doubt as to what the problem is. If there is already speech and language delay referral for a hearing assessment is required irrespective of the otoscopic findings. Otherwise, reassessment six weeks later allows the situation to be reviewed. Those with transitory middle ear fluid are most likely to have resolved by then. If

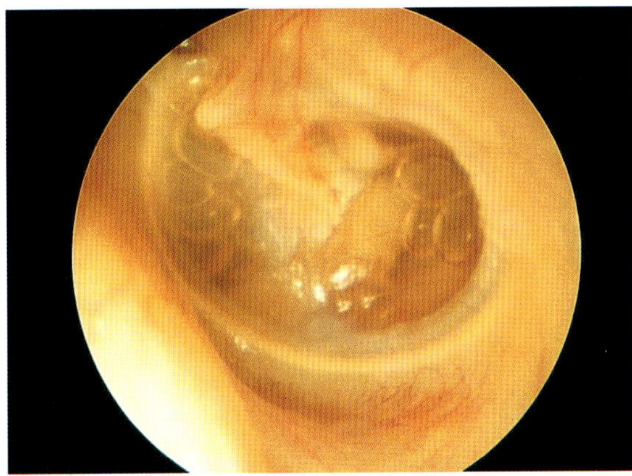

FIGURE 5.10 *Air bubbles in otitis media with effusion. Left ear.*

concern remains, a specialist opinion is required.

HOW TO DIAGNOSE OTITIS MEDIA WITH EFFUSION – SPECIALIST

The specialist has several sequential tasks:

1. Otoscopy. Confirm or exclude the diagnosis of otitis media with effusion. Otoscopy remains the key to diagnosis but this should be easier for the specialist because of the availability of pneumatic otoscopy (pages 79–80), microscopic magnification and suction to clear the canal.

   Tympanometry is of particular value when the tympanic membrane is obscured by wax. The absence of a peak between -300 and $+300\,\mathrm{mmH_2O}$ is virtually diagnostic of OME. Many would argue that even if the tympanic membrane can be seen, tympanometry should be routinely carried out because even experienced clinicians can be mistaken.

2. Assess the hearing. This is always best done by some form of audiometry. Under the age of three, distraction testing is the conventional method of doing this. Unfortunately, to get accurate thresholds requires an extremely skilled tester but the task can be made easier with visual reinforced audiometry (VRA). Children over the age of three years can almost always co-operate with pure-tone audiometry. This might initially have to be free-field rather than with headphones though most children can eventually be encouraged to wear these. The child's method of response is some form of game, such as putting pegs in a board. If a bilateral impairment is present on testing the air conduction thresholds, the not-masked bone conduction thresholds should be attempted to rule out a sensorineural impairment. This is particularly important if there is doubt otoscopically about the diagnosis of otitis media with effusion, or the tympanogram is peaked.

3. History. This is important to take for two reasons. The first is to assess the parents' degree of concern and its duration. The latter may influence how soon surgery is suggested, though it is recommended that in all a watchful waiting period is observed with a reassessment before a decision is made, because of the high chance of spontaneous resolution (Effective Health Care, 1992). The second reason for taking a history is to assess the various factors that might predict resolution. Older children and girls are less likely to have persistent fluid than younger children and boys. Because of the increased risk of upper respiratory tract infections, those at nursery or other schools are more likely to persist, as are those in smoking households and the lower socio-economic groups. Resolution is least likely in the winter.

Having done this, the specialist has to consider the aims and means of management. The insertion of ventilation tubes (grommets; Figure 5.11), with or without adenoidectomy, is the only proven management. Ventilating tubes are usually naturally extruded (Figure 5.12) though they may become non-functioning before this if they become blocked. Unfortunately ventilation tubes are associated with an increased risk of infection, both in the middle ear and around them (Figure 5.13).

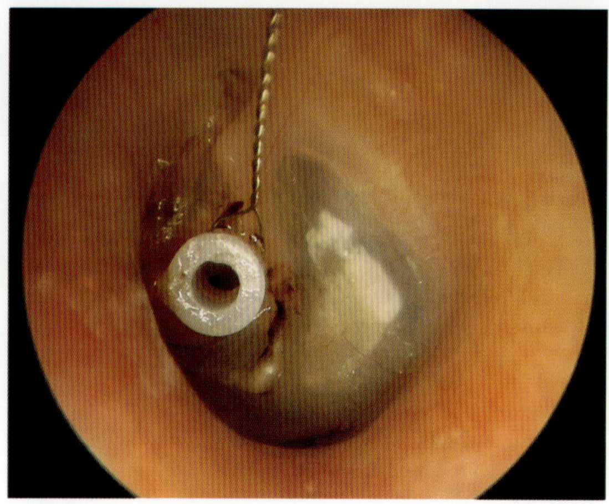

FIGURE 5.11 *Ventilating tube (grommet) placed antero-inferiorly. Left ear.*

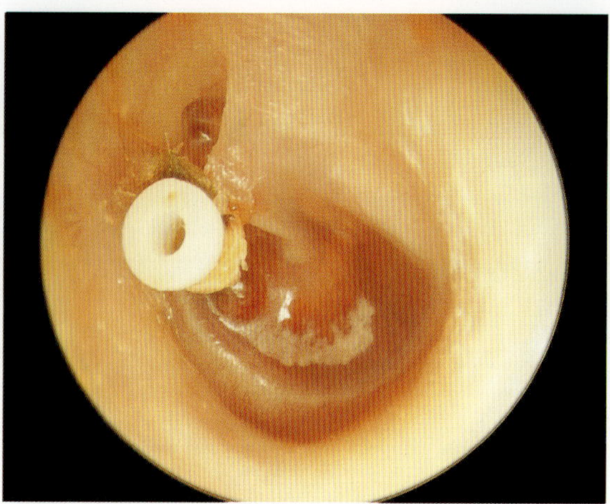

FIGURE 5.12 *Extruded ventilating tube with otoscopic recurrence of middle ear fluid. Left ear retracted and yellow.*

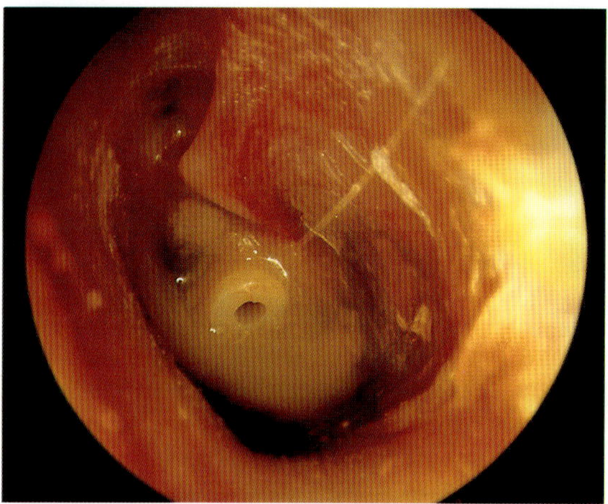

FIGURE 5.13 *Pus secondary to insertion of ventilating tube. Left ear.*

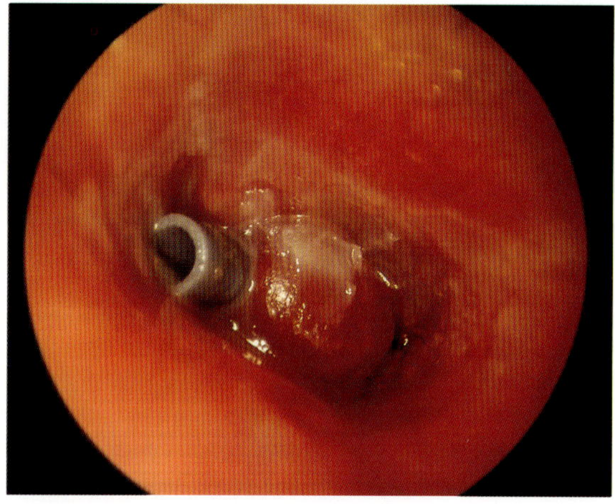

FIGURE 5.14 *Granulation tissue secondary to ventilating tube (blue, long-term tube). Left ear.*

Less commonly granulation tissue can form (Figure 5.14), particularly with long-term tubes. Unfortunately the alternatives of medical therapy including nasal decongestants, antibiotics, antihistamines and topical nasal steroids are of unproven, long-term benefit. The current opinion is that surgery should only be performed if a child has proven, bilateral OME for three months associated with an audiometric proven bilateral hearing impairment of 25 dB HL or greater. It is assumed, though by no means proven, that the speech and language delay that might occur because of prolonged hearing impairment is thereby averted. Unfortunately, there is no evidence that any therapy, including surgery, lessens the risk of the otoscopic sequelae of OME (see below). Indeed, surgery almost certainly increases the risk of tympanosclerosis, infection and chronic perforation.

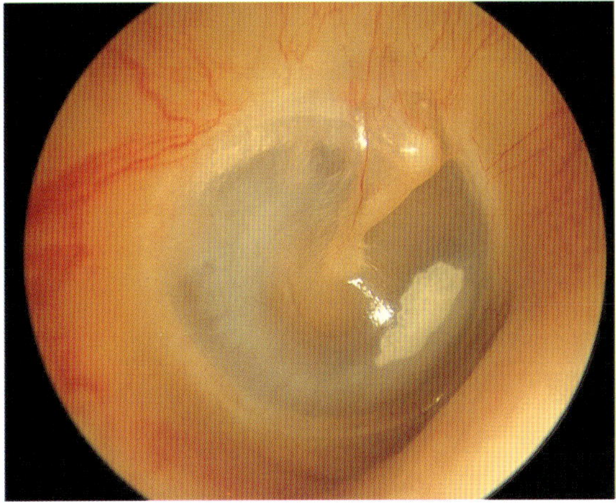

FIGURE 5.15 *Chalk patch on anterior pars tensa. Right ear.*

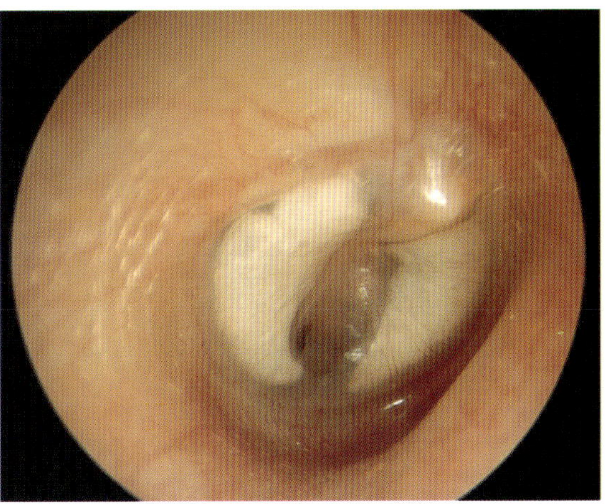

FIGURE 5.16 *Tympanosclerotic plaques, one anterior, one posterior. Right ear.*

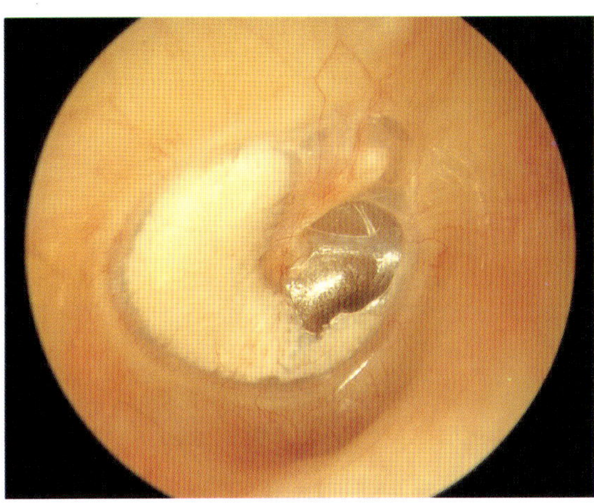

FIGURE 5.17 *Tympanosclerotic plaques, extending from posterior to inferior. Remainder of tympanic membrane scarred. Right ear.*

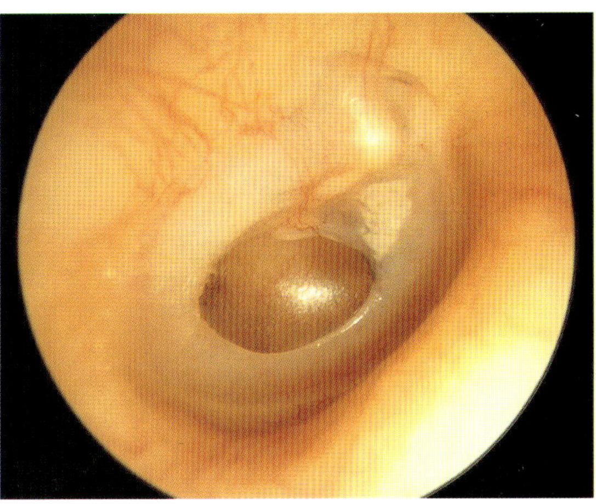

FIGURE 5.18 *Localised retraction of pars tensa affecting central area. Right ear.*

OTOLOGICAL COMPLICATIONS OF OTITIS MEDIA WITH EFFUSION

Prolonged OME, especially if surgically treated by myringotomy and insertion of grommets, is frequently associated with tympanosclerosis. In most instances this starts as chalk patches (Figure 5.15) which are of minimal concern. With time larger plaques (Figures 5.16 and 5.17) may develop which may be associated with a conductive hearing impairment in later life (see page 24). Less frequently, localised retractions of the pars tensa occur (Figure 5.18); these can be in any position but posterior ones are of particular concern because they may lead to progressive erosion of the long process of the incus and be associated with a hearing impairment (Figures 5.19 and 5.20). In addition, if

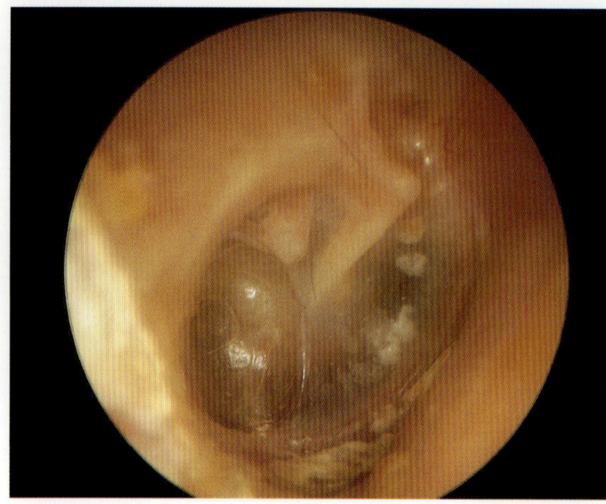

FIGURE 5.19 *Posterior retraction of tympanic membrane. Ossicular chain intact. Small anterior chalk patch. Right ear.*

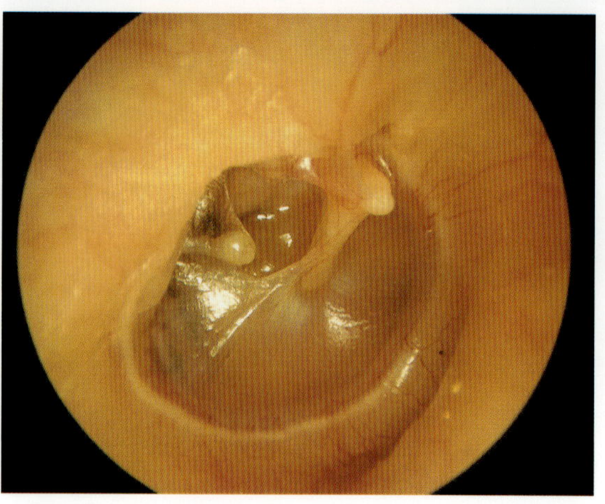

FIGURE 5.20 *Posterior retraction of tympanic membrane. Loss of long process of incus. Stapes head and tendon remain. Right ear.*

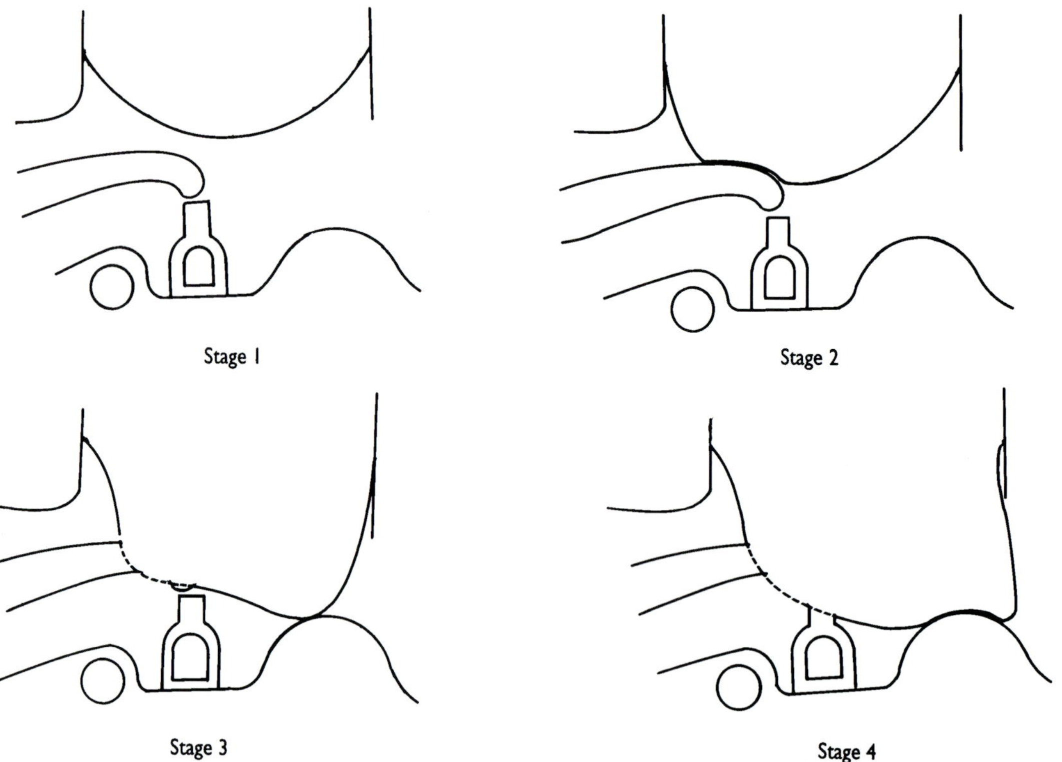

FIGURE 5.21 *Sadé and Berco's (1976) classification of retractions of pars tensa.*

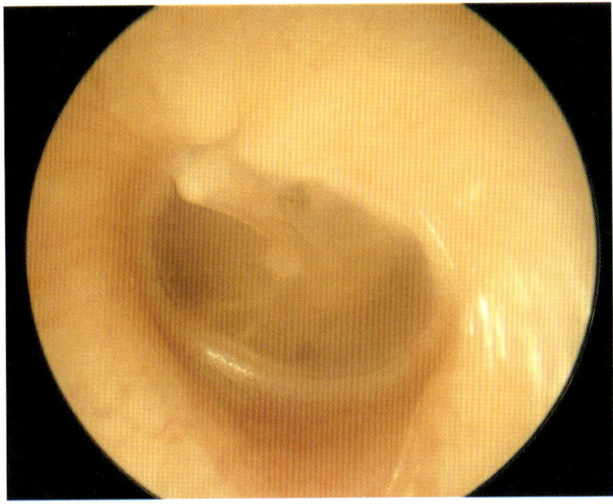

FIGURE 5.22 *Stage 1. Pars tensa retracted. There is no middle ear fluid. Left ear.*

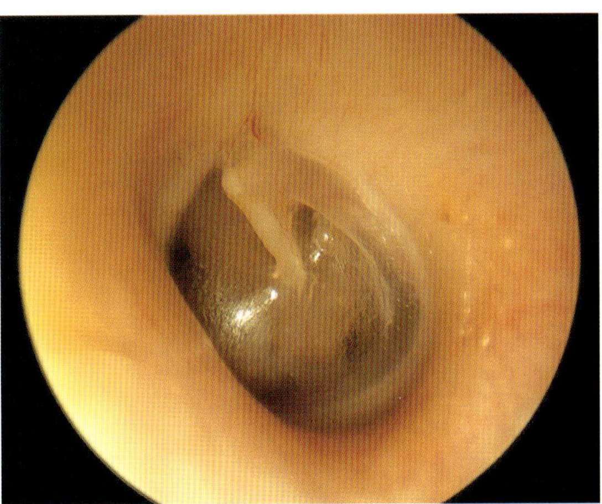

FIGURE 5.23 *Stage 2. Pars tensa severely retracted. The tympanic membrane is in contact with the long process of the incus. Left ear.*

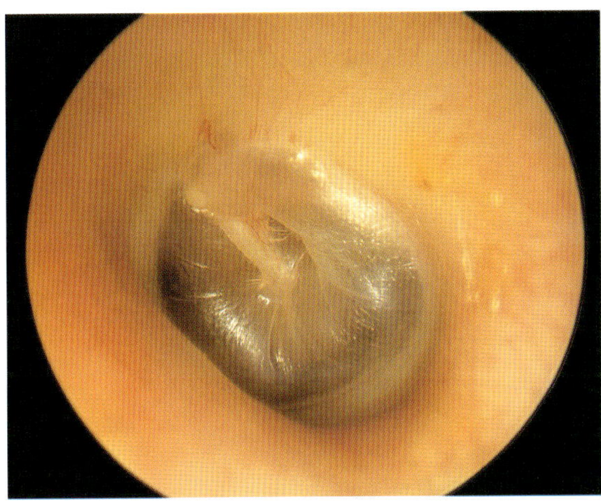

FIGURE 5.24 *Valsalva manoeuvre in same ear as Figure 5.23 demonstrating that the tympanic membrane is adherent to the long process of the incus.*

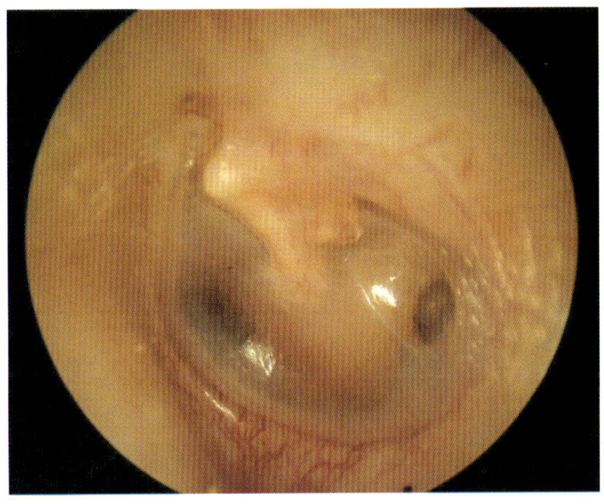

FIGURE 5.25 *Stage 3. Atelectasis. Tympanic membrane retracted on to promontory. Left ear.*

retraction progresses posterosuperiorly then it may progress to active squamous COM – a cholesteatoma. Hence, whenever a retraction is identified, referral to a specialist is required.

Pars tensa retraction – specialist

Pars tensa retractions have been classified by Sadé and Berco (1976) into four stages (Figure 5.21). The distinction between them can be difficult and often depends on whether the retracted membrane is adherent to the ossicles or promontory. To assess whether this is the case, the ear is observed whilst the patient performs a Valsalva manoeuvre. Often the patient cannot do this and the mobility has to be otherwise assessed by pneumatic otoscopy.

Retractions can affect a variable proportion of the pars tensa but they most frequently affect the posterior part. This is of particular concern because of the anatomy of this area.

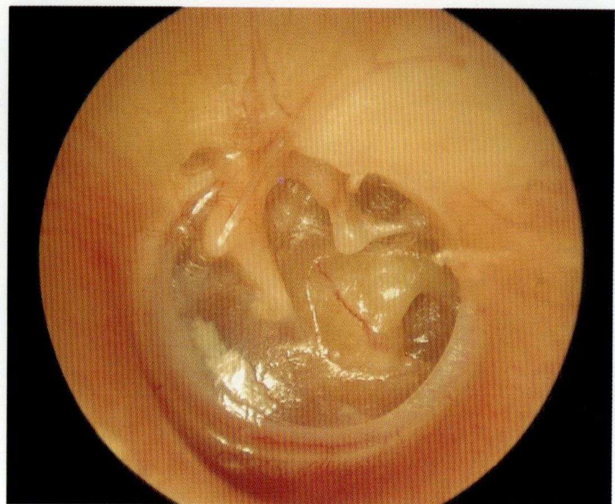

FIGURE 5.26 *Stage 4.* Adhesive otitis. *The pars tensa is adherent to the promontory and draped around the long process of the incus and stapes. Left ear.*

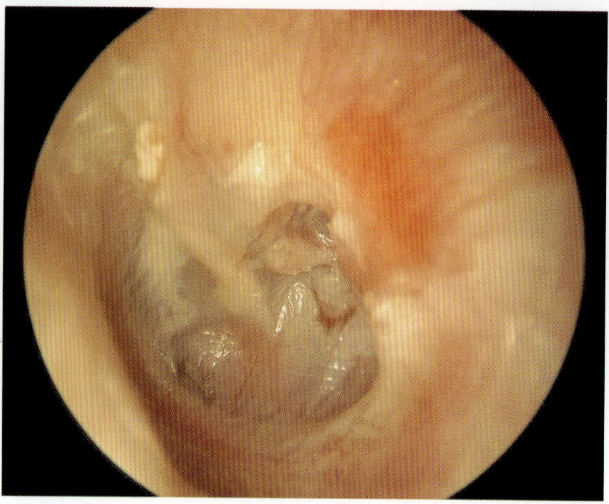

FIGURE 5.27 *Posterior atelectatic pars tensa. The long process of the incus is necrosed and the posterior part of the retraction is out of view. A small area of granulation on posterior canal indicates activity and early cholesteatoma. Left ear.*

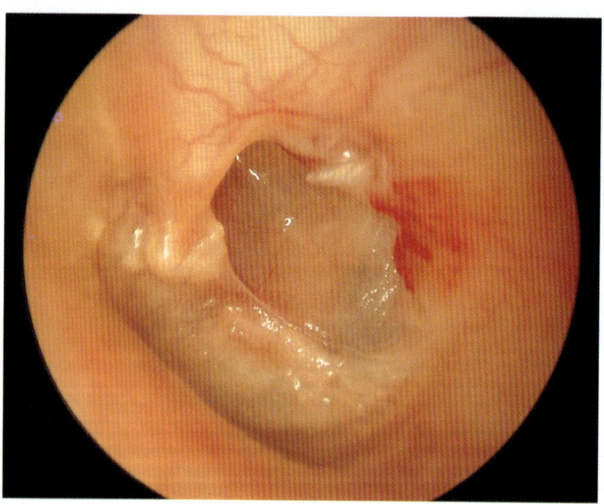

FIGURE 5.28 *Posterior atelectatic pars tensa with erosion of posterior canal wall as well as long process of incus and stapes superstructure. Prominent granulations on posterior canal wall suggestive of progressive cholesteatoma for Figure 5.27. Left ear.*

The ossicular chain in particular can create a retraction that is out of vision with a narrow neck. In some this gives rise to active (squamous) COM – a cholesteatoma.

Stage 1 – Slight retraction
Distinguishing a slight degree of retraction (Figure 5.22) from a normal ear (Figure 5.2) can be difficult. A foreshortened appearance of the malleus handle and lipping of the tympanic membrane at the annulus should be looked for. The tympanic membrane is not in contact with the incus or stapes and is mobile on pneumatic otoscopy which also excludes coexisting middle ear fluid.

Stage 2 – severe retraction
The tympanic membrane is retracted onto the long process of the incus or the stapes and may or may not be adherent to them. Figures 5.23 and 5.24 are examples where on a Valsalva manoeuvre the tympanic membrane is adherent to the ossicles.

Stage 3 – atelectasis
The tympanic membrane is even more retracted and is in contact with, but not adherent to, the promontory. Figure 5.25 is an example where the tympanic membrane is in contact with the promontory but not adherent on a Valsalva manoeuvre.

Stage 4 – adhesive otitis
The retracted tympanic membrane is adherent to the promontory (Figure 5.26).

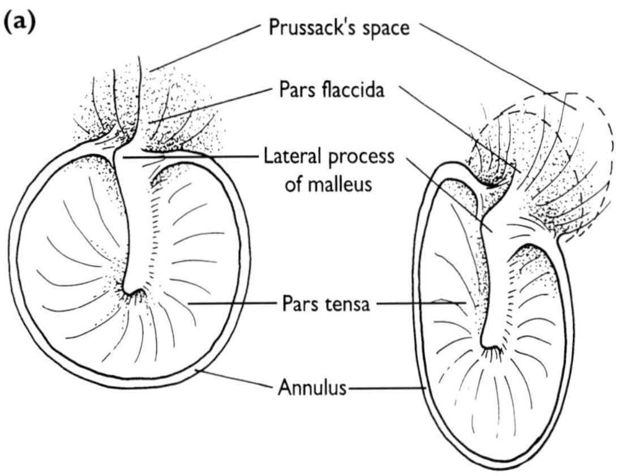

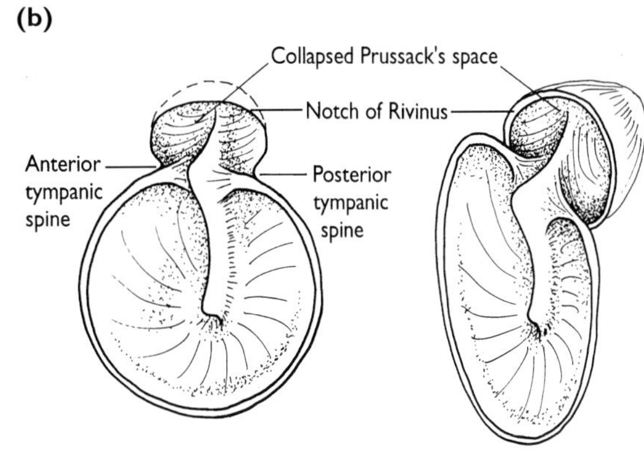

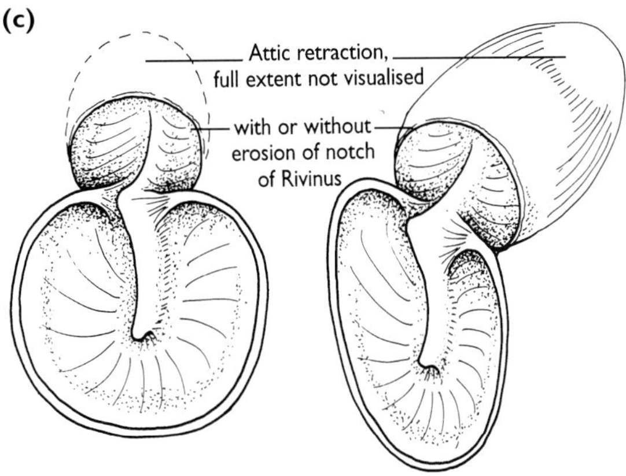

FIGURE 5.29 *Left ear viewed otoscopically from slightly different angles. (a) Drawing of normal epitympanum to show Prussack's space. (b) Early pars flaccida retraction (Tos II). (c) Marked pars flaccida retraction (Tos III and IV).*

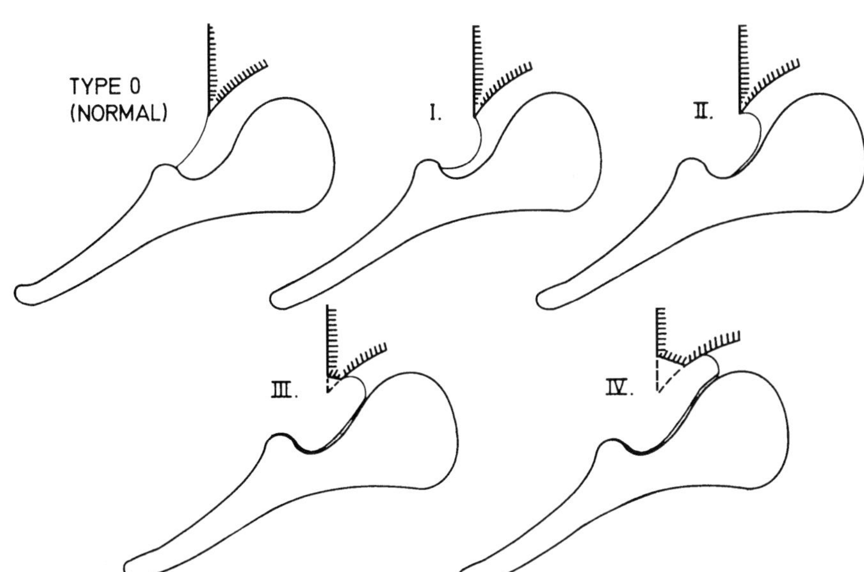

FIGURE 5.30
Drawing after Tos et al. (1987) of classification of pars flaccida retractions, grades 0–IV. Coronal section of the left ear seen from behind. Pars flaccida is the membrane between the lateral process of the malleus and the bony attic wall (hatched). As the pars flaccida becomes more retracted, the pocket becomes more out of view and the bony attic wall may become eroded (grades III and IV).

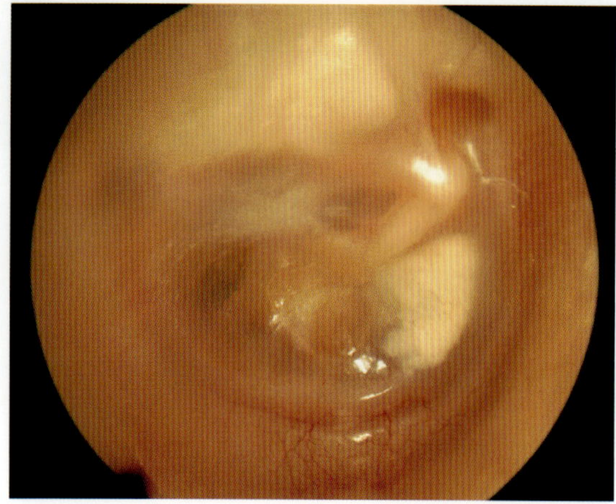

FIGURE 5.31 *Stage 1 retraction of pars flaccida. Simple attic dimple. Coincident anterior tympanosclerotic patch of pars tensa. Right ear.*

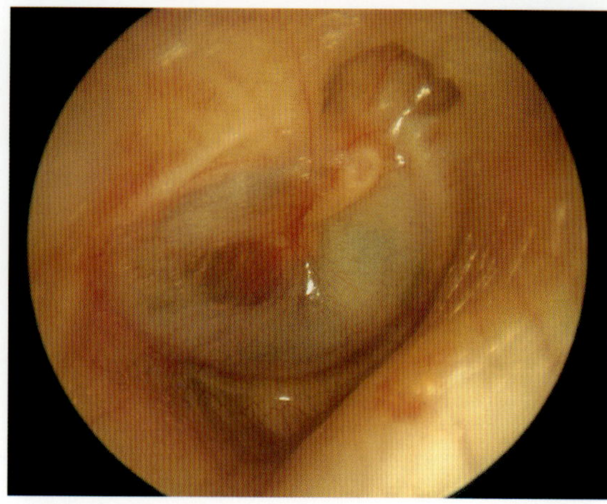

FIGURE 5.32 *Stage 2 retraction of pars flaccida. Retraction adherent to neck of malleus. Right ear.*

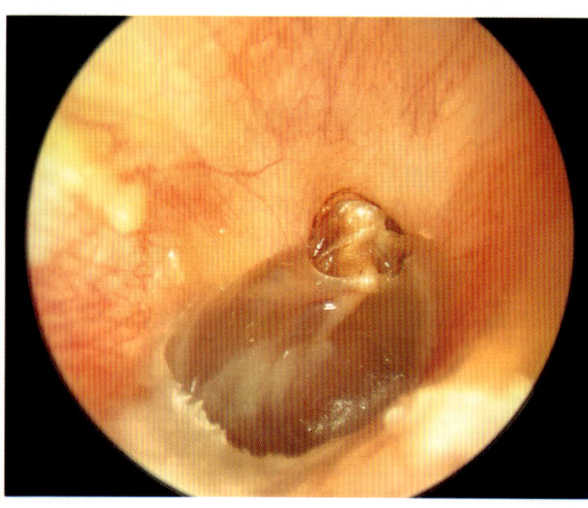

FIGURE 5.33 *Stage 3 retraction of pars flaccida. Part of retraction out of view. Suggestion of middle ear fluid. Right ear.*

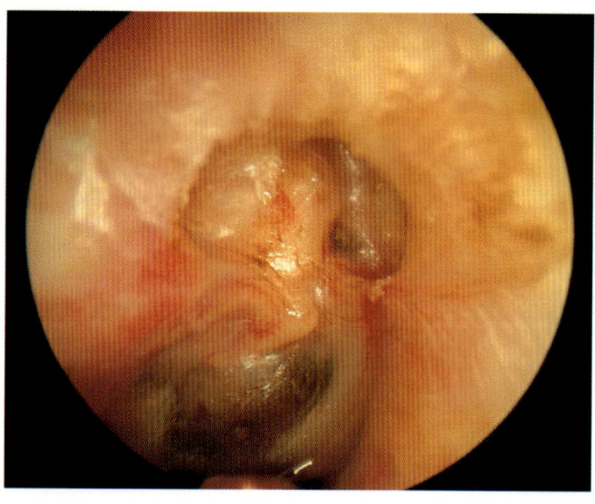

FIGURE 5.34 *Stage 4 retraction of pars flaccida. Erosion of bony attic wall and part of retraction out of view. No activity. Right ear.*

Management

Many consider retractions should be energetically managed to prevent necrosis of the long process of the incus and the development of a middle ear cholesteatoma (active squamous COM). This is more likely with posterior retractions and is often first detected by the appearance of granulation tissue on the posterior canal wall (Figures 5.27 and 5.28). Unfortunately ventilating tubes (grommets) have no long-term effect on retraction pockets even in Stages 1 and 2 where there are no adhesions. Many now advocate removal of the retraction pocket, some leaving it to heal spontaneously whilst others perform a myringoplasty.

Pars flaccida retraction – specialist

Retractions of the pars flaccida without involvement or abnormality of the pars tensa occur

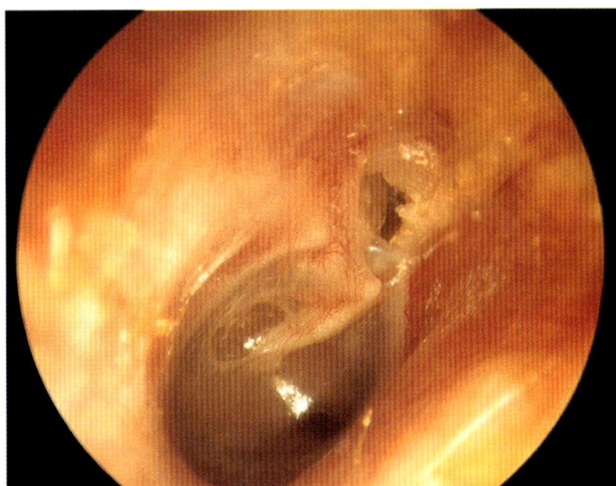

FIGURE 5.35 *Attic retraction as figure 5.33 but with retention of squamous epithelial debris and secondary activity. Right ear.*

due to poor aeration of the epitympanum, specifically of Prussack's space (Figure 5.29). Communication between the epitympanum and mesotympanum is limited by mucosal folds around the ossicular chain. Mucosal oedema may stenose these openings and lead to poor aeration and chronic disease of the attic. Chronic negative pressure in Prussack's space may result in its roof, i.e. the pars flaccida, collapsing onto its floor.

Tos *et al.* (1987) have described four distinct stages of attic retraction (Figure 5.30). In Stage 1 the pars flaccida is a dimple which is more retracted than normal but not adherent to the neck of the malleus (Figure 5.31). In Stage 2 the retraction is adherent to the neck of the malleus but the entire extent of the retraction pocket can be seen (Figure 5.32). In Stage 3, part of the retraction pocket cannot be seen and there may be partial erosion of the bony attic wall (Figure 5.33). In Stage 4 there is definite bony erosion of the attic with the extent of the retraction being uncertain because it is out of vision (Figure 5.34).

In Stages 1 and 2 the retractions are, in general, self-cleansing. However, in Stages 3 and 4 squamous debris may accumulate and become active squamous COM – a cholesteatoma. The distinction between a self-cleaning retraction pocket and a cholesteatoma is sometimes difficult because the accumulated debris may be out of sight. The presence of epithelial debris (Figure 5.35), pus or crusting is diagnostic of an established cholesteatoma.

Management

It is usual to follow up children with retraction pockets to ensure that if a cholesteatoma develops it is identified early. However, the chances of this occurring in Stages 1, 2 and 3 are extremely low and there is no proven way, including the insertion of ventilating tubes, of preventing cholesteatoma developing.

CHAPTER 6

THE PAINFUL EAR

Pain in and around the ear (otalgia) is a relatively common symptom in children and adults. The more likely causes are different in each of these age groups though the mechanisms by which pain occurs are identical.

Otalgia can either be otological or non-otological in origin. The sensory supply of the skin of the pinna and of the external auditory canal is a combination of cervical nerves C2 and C3, the trigeminal (V), facial (VII) and vagus (X) cranial nerves (Figure 6.1). The mucosa of the middle ear is supplied by the glossopharyngeal (IX) nerve. All these nerves supply other areas of the head and neck and, because localisation is not particularly good, pain in the ear can be referred from pathology elsewhere. Such referred pain is particularly likely to occur in structures supplied by the Vth and IXth cranial nerves. Another reason that otalgia can be non-otological in origin is that it arises in structures close to the ear. Such structures include the temporomandibular joint, the parotid gland and the cervical spine.

Pain that originates in the ear can be one of two main types depending on whether the skin or the middle ear is involved. To make this distinction is particularly helpful in adults. Skin conditions, particularly otitis externa, cause an irritative discomfort making the patient wish to poke the ear. Middle ear disease causes a much sharper pain, mainly due to acute changes in pressure across the tympanic membrane. Thus otalgia is common during aeroplane flights when there is an acute pressure difference at the tympanic membrane between the external environment and the middle ear. By comparison chronic pressure differences across the tympanic membrane are usually not painful.

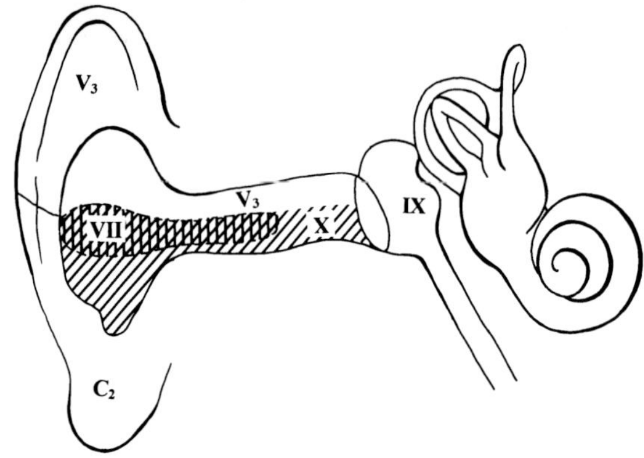

FIGURE 6.1 *Sensory nerve supply of the external and middle ear. C_2 = Cervical C2 and 3. V_3 = Mandibular branch of trigeminal nerve. VII = Facial nerve. IX = Glossopharyngeal nerve. X = Vagus nerve.*

Otoscopy will distinguish otologic from non-otologic causes because the former all cause otoscopic abnormalities. If the ear is normal, non-otologic causes have to be sought. Table 6.1 lists the main otological and non-otological causes of otalgia in children and adults. The non-otological causes are not discussed in detail. Some of the otological causes are discussed in greater detail in other chapters because the dominant symptom is not otalgia.

OTALGIA IN CHILDREN

Acute otitis media is the most common, painful ear condition of childhood, though its presen-

TABLE 6.1 *Causes of otalgia*

Conditions	Children	Adults
Otologic	**Acute otitis media***	**Furuncle***
	Otitis externa*	**Otitis externa***
	Foreign body*	**Barotrauma**
	Otitis media with effusion	Herpes zoster*
	Acute mastoiditis	Bullous myringitis*
		Acute otitis media*
		Carcinoma of middle ear
Non-otologic	**Teething**	**Cervical osteoarthritis**
	Upper respiratory infection	**Temporomandibular joint**
	Pharyngitis	**Parotitis**
	Tonsillitis	**Unerupted molars**
	Caries	**Pharyngitis**
		Carcinoma of base of tongue
		Carcinoma of pharynx

Conditions in non-bold typeface are uncommon diagnoses.
**Conditions illustrated in this chapter.*

tation differs with age. In infants up to nine months of age, AOM normally presents with non-specific irritability, poor feeding and pyrexia. If otoscopy is normal, teething is the most frequent non-otologic cause of such a group of symptoms but other infections, such as in the chest or urinary tract, have also to be considered. In those between nine months and three years of age the most common history is of waking up at night, pulling or holding the ear. There is frequently a preceding upper respiratory tract infection. Again, if otoscopy is normal, teething is the most common cause of referred pain but pharyngitis and tonsillitis associated with a respiratory tract infection may also be the cause. Over the age of three years, the child is likely to report that their ear is sore. In them, dental caries and upper respiratory tract infections remain common causes of referred pain.

At all ages, the clinician needs to obtain and maintain the child's confidence when examining the ears. Once the child becomes scared and unco-operative, successful diagnosis is less likely. Part of the problem is as soon as the child starts to struggle or cry, there is decreased blood flow from the head and neck because of venous stasis. A tympanic flush then develops which may mistakenly be diagnosed as AOM. Irritation from attempted and repeated use of an aural speculum also causes a tympanic flush.

Look at summary tree 6.1

In most children, otoscopy ① should give at least a partial view of the tympanic membrane. If it does not ②, wax and foreign bodies are easily identifiable reasons. Otitis externa only becomes likely in older children.

FOREIGN BODIES

Foreign bodies are not infrequently placed in the external canal by young children (Figure 6.2). They can remain symptom free for some time, and then present because of secondary otitis externa. Diagnosis is straightforward and management is their removal, usually by syringing.

OTITIS EXTERNA

In children, otitis externa most frequently follows swimming, particularly in hot, humid climates, and is exacerbated by poking the ear with various instruments. The clinical findings and management are as for adults (see page 48).

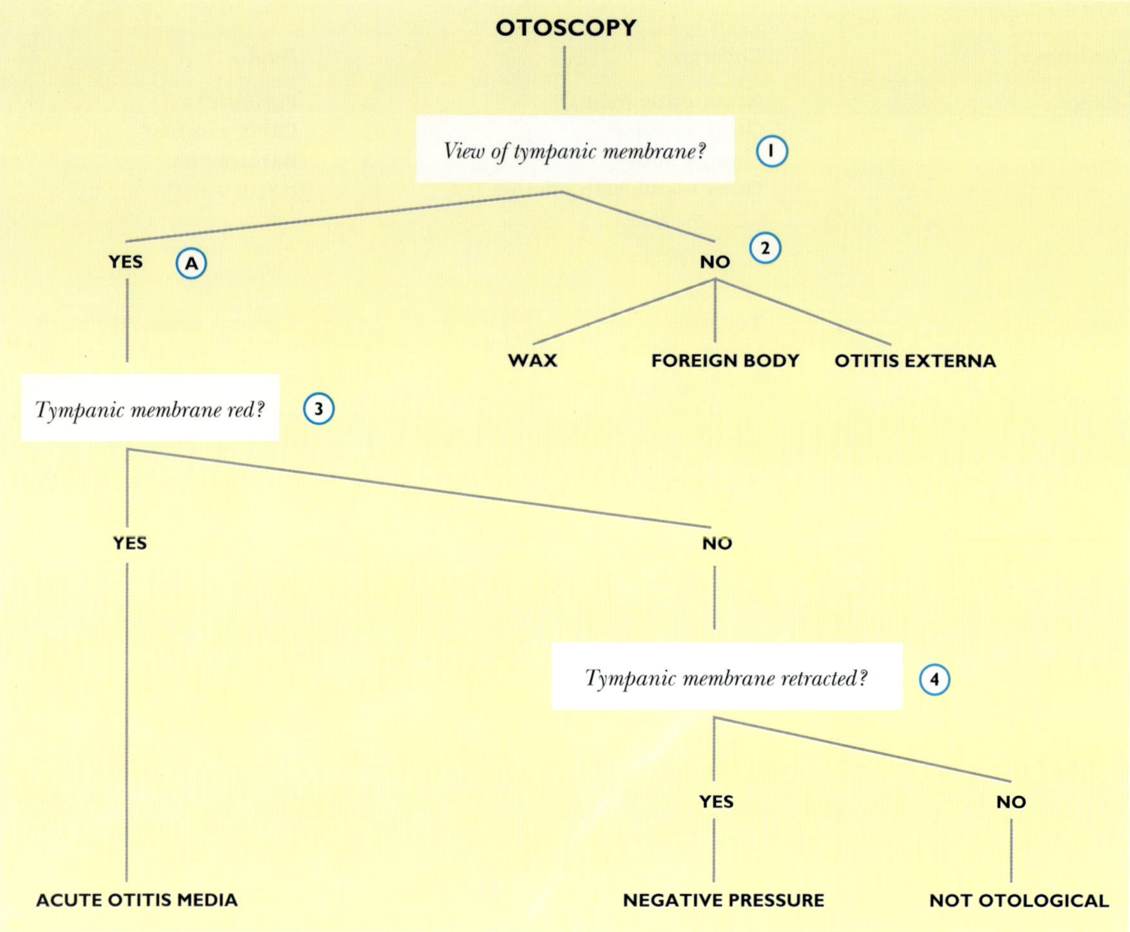

OTOSCOPY

View of tympanic membrane? ①

YES Ⓐ   NO ②

WAX   FOREIGN BODY   OTITIS EXTERNA

Tympanic membrane red? ③

YES   NO

Tympanic membrane retracted? ④

YES   NO

ACUTE OTITIS MEDIA   NEGATIVE PRESSURE   NOT OTOLOGICAL

Summary tree 6.1 Otalgia in children.

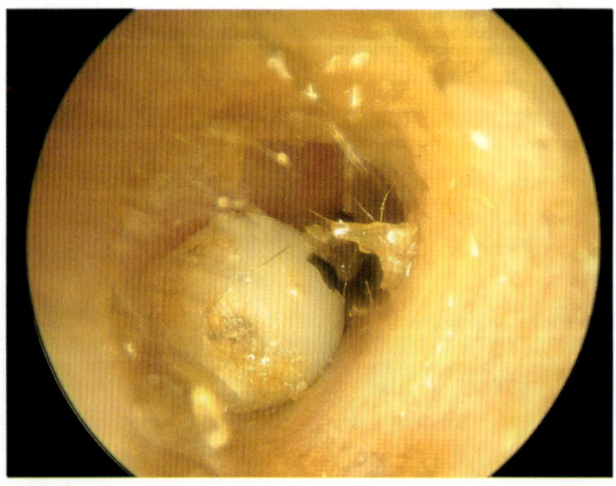

FIGURE 6.2 *Foreign body in right external auditory canal.*

Look at branch 6.1A

Having excluded canal pathology and identified the tympanic membrane, the first thing to assess is its degree of redness ③ and whether it bulges. The main diagnosis to consider is AOM.

ACUTE OTITIS MEDIA

Acute otitis media has several stages. Early on, the canal is normal but the blood vessels along the handle of the malleus and the edge of the tympanic membrane become prominent (Figure 6.3). The tympanic membrane loses its translucency and becomes dull and red (Figure 6.4). Progressively the tympanic membrane and

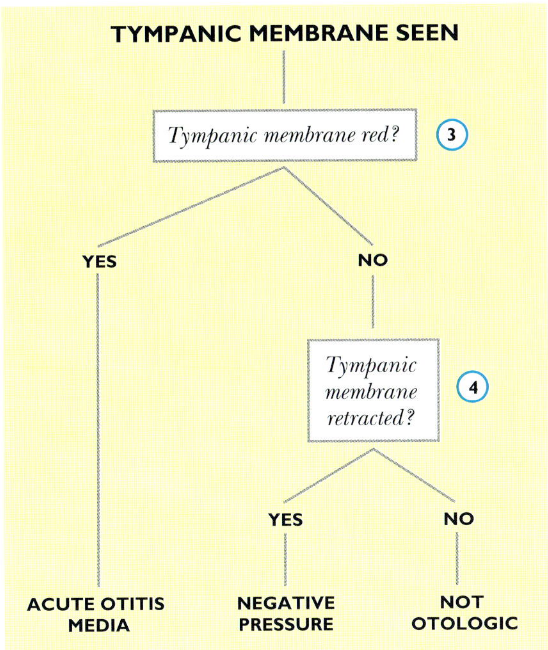

Branch 6.1A

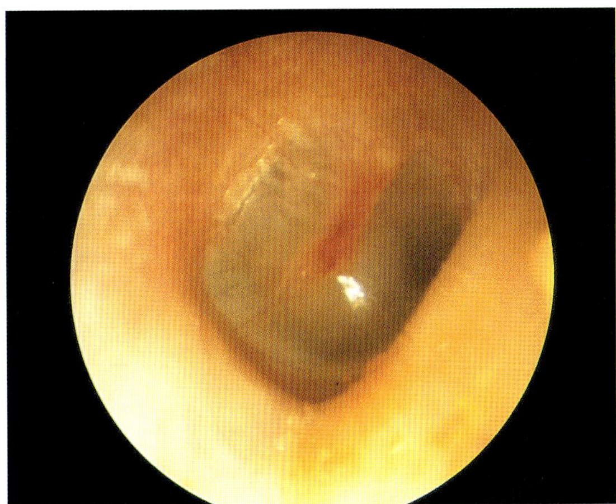

FIGURE 6.3 *Early (right) acute otitis media showing prominent blood vessels. Tympanic membrane essentially normal.*

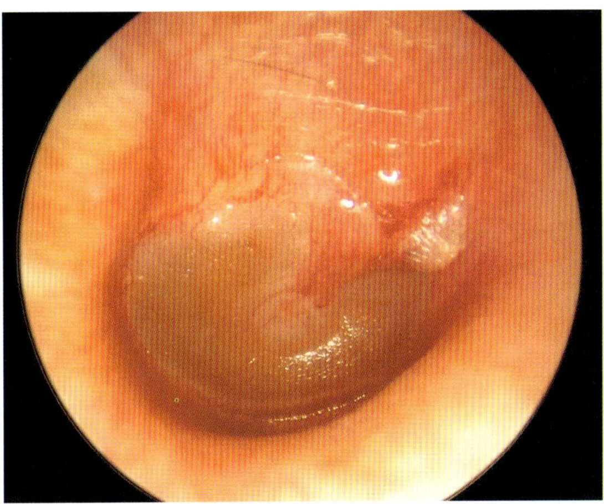

FIGURE 6.4 *Mid-stage acute otitis media (right). Tympanic membrane becomes red and loses translucency.*

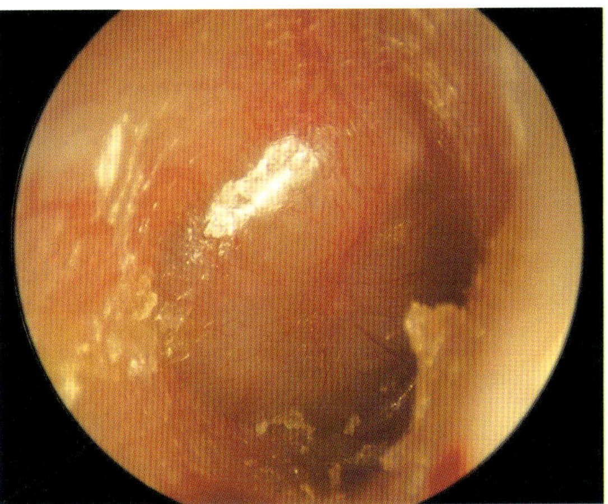

FIGURE 6.5 *Late acute otitis media (right). Bulging red tympanic membrane.*

surrounding skin of the deep external auditory canal become inflamed. The tympanic membrane bulges out under pressure from pus in the middle ear (Figure 6.5). In some a small perforation then occurs through which pus is discharged (Figure 6.6). This usually relieves the otalgia.

Management

As the child has a sore ear, analgesics are the mainstay of management. The indications for antibiotics are controversial. Symptomatically the majority (80%) of children with AOM will settle spontaneously within 48 hours, so many consider that antibiotics should be reserved for

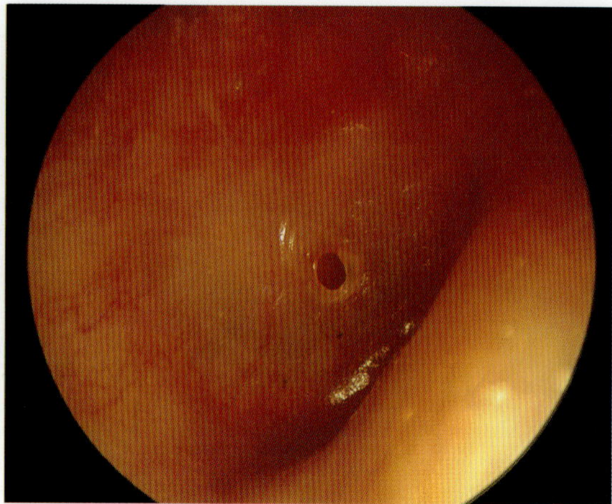

FIGURE 6.6 *Pinhole perforation in acute otitis media. Right ear.*

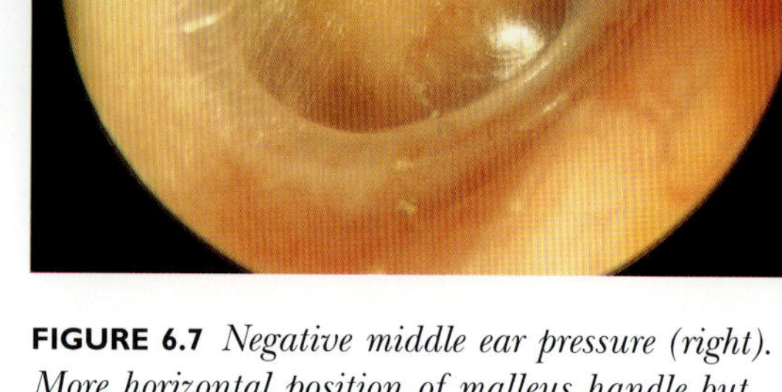

FIGURE 6.7 *Negative middle ear pressure (right). More horizontal position of malleus handle but normal colour of tympanic membrane.*

those that have not settled by that time. Obviously, prior to that, if a child is systemically unwell then antibiotics should be prescribed. The antibiotic of choice is amoxycillin.

Children who have had AOM should all be followed up because about 10% will still have middle ear fluid 12 weeks later which is perhaps associated with a hearing impairment. They then need to be managed as a child with OME.

If the symptoms of AOM do not settle after three days of antibiotic therapy then referral to a specialist is suggested, because it is this group that may develop meningitis or acute mastoiditis.

Acute otitis media – specialist

In many countries, children with otalgia are initially seen by a paediatrician or an otolaryngologist rather than a primary care physician. The decision process whereby a specialist arrives at a diagnosis is understandably more complicated and takes several interacting aspects into account, apart from the fact that the ear is red. The alternative diagnoses to consider are a red tympanic flush due to crying or fever, and a dull pars tensa, often seen in otitis media with effusion.

Laterality of red ear

The majority of children with a red ear due to crying or fever will have bilateral otoscopic redness. On the other hand, less than a quarter (25%) of children with proven AOM will have it bilaterally.

Position of tympanic membrane

As purulent fluid progressively collects in the middle ear, the tympanic membrane not only becomes redder but bulges.

Mobility of tympanic membrane

Assessing the mobility of the tympanic membrane by pneumatic otoscopy is perhaps the most useful additional assessment that can be done, provided it is practicable. A mobile tympanic membrane virtually excludes acute otitis media.

ACUTE MASTOIDITIS

Very rarely (0.01%) AOM progresses to acute mastoiditis. This is usually suspected by continued illness with septicaemia. Otoscopy shows the classical signs of an acutely inflamed, nondraining, bulging tympanic membrane. There is postauricular induration because of infection trapped within the mastoid air cells and sometimes there is a subperiosteal abscess. Systemic antibiotics and surgical drainage are crucial.

Look at branch 6.1A

In non-reddened tympanic membranes, a decision has to be made whether it is retracted

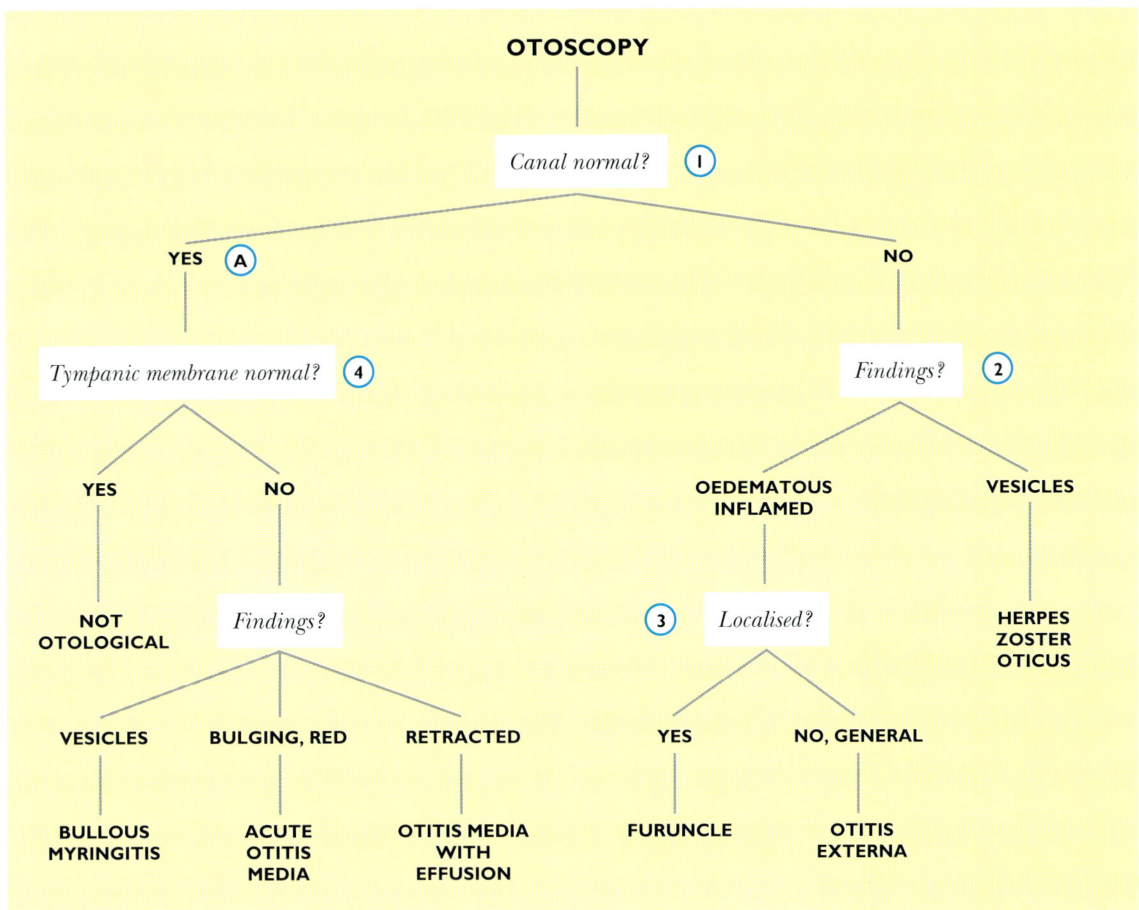

Summary tree 6.2 Otalgia in adults.

or not ④. The most likely diagnosis is negative middle ear pressure; OME is less likely. If the tympanic membrane is not retracted, non-otologic causes should be looked for.

NEGATIVE MIDDLE EAR PRESSURE

Painful negative middle ear pressure occurs because of absorption of the middle ear gases which cannot be compensated for because of the poor Eustachian tube function associated with an upper respiratory tract infection. The handle of the malleus takes a more horizontal position (Figure 6.7) but the tympanic membrane will still move on pneumatic otoscopy. Its colour is normal which helps distinguish it from OME.

OTITIS MEDIA WITH EFFUSION

The majority of children with OME do not have otalgia. However, there may be a history of otalgia in those in whom an episode of AOM was the initiating factor. The diagnosis of OME is discussed on pages 30–34.

OTALGIA IN ADULTS

Acute otitis media is primarily a condition of those under ten years of age. Above that age other diagnoses, particularly otitis externa, become more likely. In the following discussion, an adult is taken as being ten years and above.

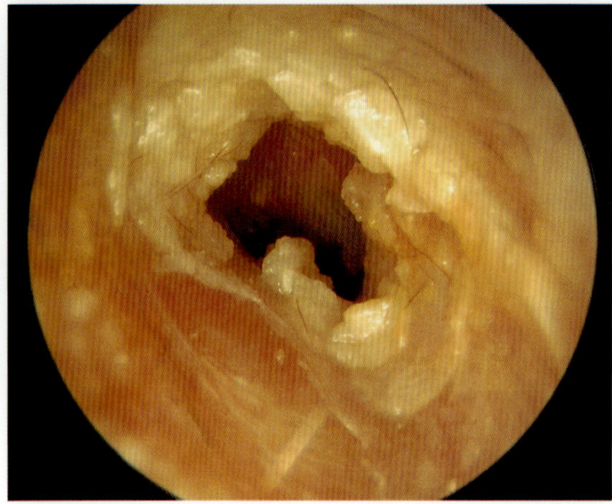

FIGURE 6.8 *Gross debris in left external auditory canal which after removal reveals otitis externa (Figure 6.9).*

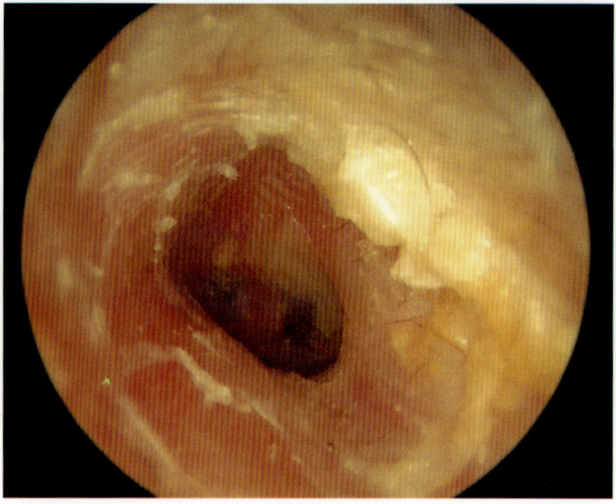

FIGURE 6.9 *Otitis externa (left). The canal skin is swollen and inflamed.*

Look at summary tree 6.2

In adults, otalgia is most frequently due to conditions of the external auditory canal, so this should be examined carefully ①. Each condition that causes canal abnormalities ② has fairly specific findings.

OTITIS EXTERNA

Otitis externa is the diagnosis if after removal of gross debris (Figure 6.8) the canal skin is generally ③ swollen and inflamed (Figure 6.9). Most frequently there is an itchy, irritative discomfort rather than a throbbing ache. The canal skin usually weeps but a discharge is not always noticed.

Otoscopy may cause discomfort, and after removal of debris in the milder cases, the canal skin will be glazed, redder than normal and perhaps slightly oedematous. The oedema increases with the condition's severity (Figure 6.10). In the most severe cases even a small aural speculum can be difficult to insert.

Management

As there is usually considerable debris when the patient is first seen, the canal is gently cleared by syringing and mopped dry (pages 83–84). This is often all that is necessary to allow mild

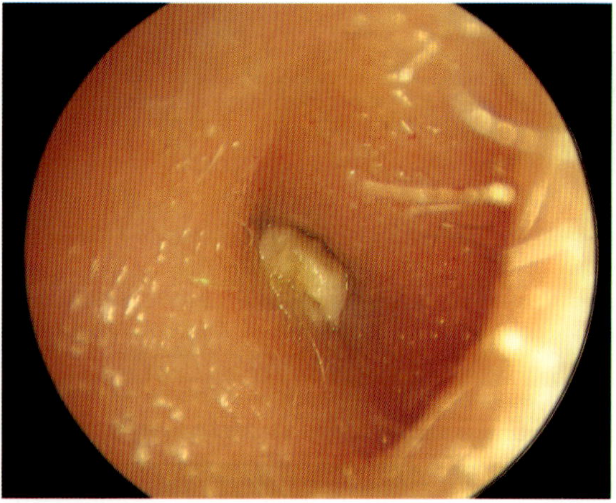

FIGURE 6.10 *Marked otitis externa (left). Canal is very narrow with retained debris.*

otitis externa to settle. If it does not, regular mopping with instillation of topical medications is instituted. The medications may be in the form of drops, sprays or ointments and usually contain a steroid (hydrocortisone, betamethasone or dexamethasone). Some clinicians include an antibiotic but care should be taken with combined medications, as antibiotics may cause allergic skin reactions. They may also

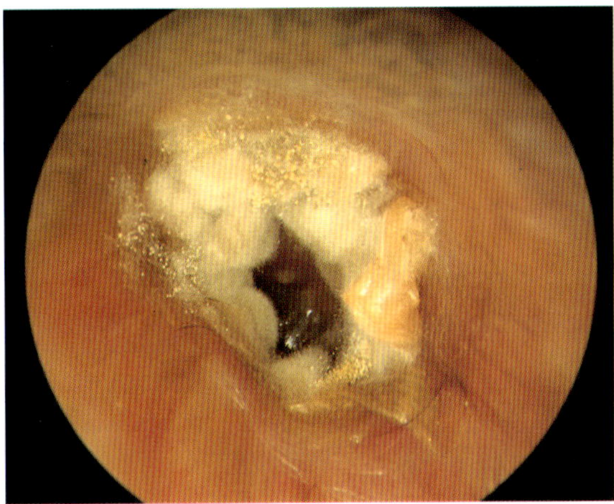

FIGURE 6.11 *Fungal otitis externa (left) with* Aspergillus flavus.

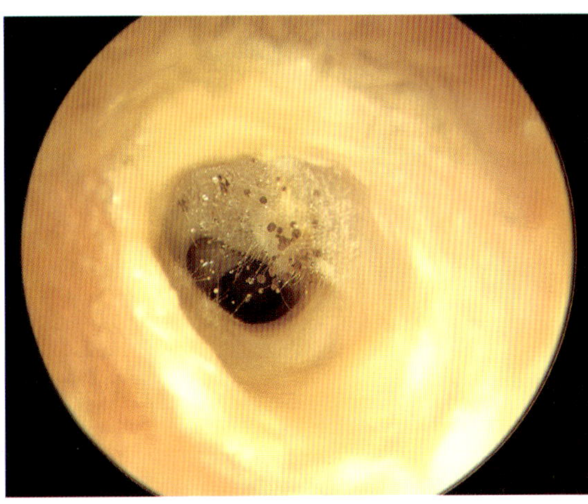

FIGURE 6.12 *Fungal otitis externa (left) with* Aspergillus niger.

encourage the growth of commensals and secondary invaders such as fungi. Hence they may worsen the condition.

The decision as to the type of preparation to use depends on the severity of the otitis externa and the patient's manual dexterity. Drops require that the head be held with the ear uppermost. It is easier for someone else to put in the correct number of drops in the canal when in this position. The tragus is then pressed several times to close the canal to ensure displacement of the drops down the canal skin. Sprays are easier for the patient to use themselves, do not require specific positioning of the head, but do require that the canal is fairly open. If the canal is considerably narrowed by oedema, a solution-laden wick should be placed in the canal and thereafter regularly kept moist with drops. These wicks require changing daily or on alternate days.

Non-response to treatment is most often due to inadequate clearing of debris from the canal. Meticulous cleaning of the canal is often difficult without suction and referral to a specialist may be necessary. An alternative reason for non-response is the development of an irritant or allergic reaction.

Otitis externa – specialist

Fungal otitis externa

Fungal overgrowth often occurs after long-term use of antibiotic and steroid drops which disturbs the normal flora of the canal. The diagnosis is not difficult, the canal being coated with hyphae with spores at their end. The most common fungi are *Aspergillus flavus* (Figure 6.11) and *Aspergillus niger* (Figure 6.12). The distinction is not important as the condition rapidly responds to meticulously removing the fungi and ceasing topical antibiotic therapy.

Malignant otitis externa

Otitis externa can become more destructive (malignant otitis externa). This should be suspected if more severe pain develops, particularly in an immunocompromised individual such as a diabetic. Pathologically there is a spreading periosteitis initially of the canal wall. If uncontrolled it spreads to the mastoid and can be associated with a facial palsy. In more 'malignant' cases, it can spread to the petrous apex and cause lower cranial nerve palsies (X, XI and XII). *Pseudomonas aeruginosa* is the organism most frequently responsible.

On otoscopy, there are granulations (Figure 6.13) and sometimes ulcers in the canal. CT

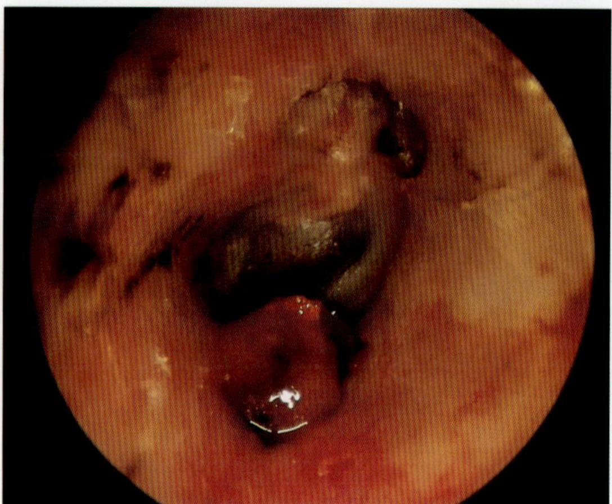

FIGURE 6.13 *Malignant otitis externa (right) with granulation tissue on the floor of the external auditory canal.*

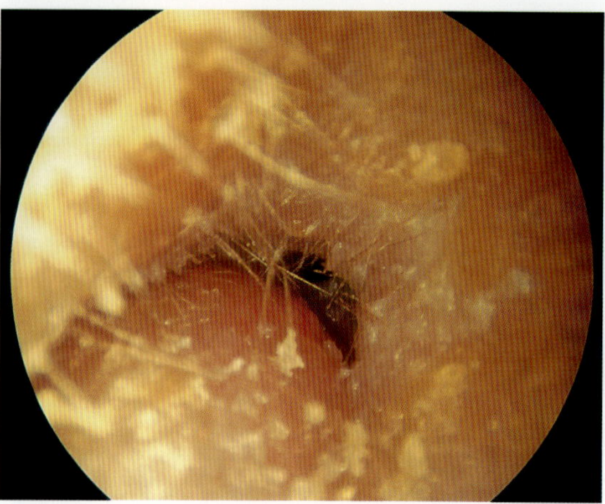

FIGURE 6.14 *Furuncle of right external auditory canal. Localised – rather than the generalised oedema of otitis externa.*

scanning should delineate the extent of bone involvement. Management is with systemic antibiotics and extensive surgical debridement of necrotic bone.

Look at summary tree 6.2 ③

FURUNCLE

Furuncles (boils) of the hair follicles of the canal skin are evident because of the localised ③ (Figure 6.14) rather than generalised canal oedema of otitis externa. Furuncles can be particularly painful, so touching the skin with an auriscope causes extreme discomfort. Management is with systemic, anti-staphylococcal antibiotics.

HERPES ZOSTER OTICUS

Here the pain is of sudden onset and intense in areas supplied by the particular nerves that are infected with herpes. A day or two later this is followed by the development of vesicles which can break down, bleed (Figure 6.15) and crust. The vesicles are mainly on the auricle and external auditory canal. In some patients a facial palsy develops before the vesicles and less

commonly there can be a hearing loss and vertigo. Treatment is primarily supportive, with pain relief until natural resolution occurs. Steroids and acyclovir can be given, if the condition is detected early, to hasten resolution.

Look at branch 6.2A

If the external auditory canal is normal, the tympanic membrane is identified and inspected. The diagnosis rests upon the findings ④.

BULLOUS MYRINGITIS

This is an acute viral infection of the tympanic membrane resulting in the formation of bullae (Figure 6.16). If these rupture, a watery blood-stained discharge may occur. Spontaneous resolution occurs between three and seven days. Treatment is symptomatic with analgesics and, if necessary, topical anaesthetic (benzocaine) ear drops.

ACUTE OTITIS MEDIA

The otoscopic appearance of AOM in adults is similar to that in older children, classically with a red, bulging drum (page 45). In adults, AOM is a relatively uncommon diagnosis.

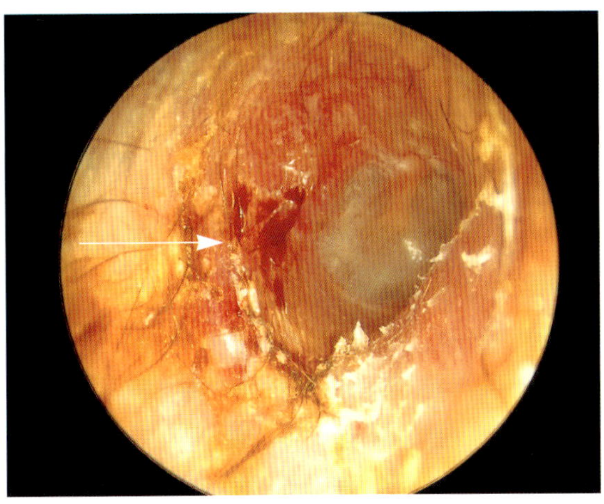

FIGURE 6.15 *Haemorrhagic vesicle of herpes zoster (arrowed). Right ear.*

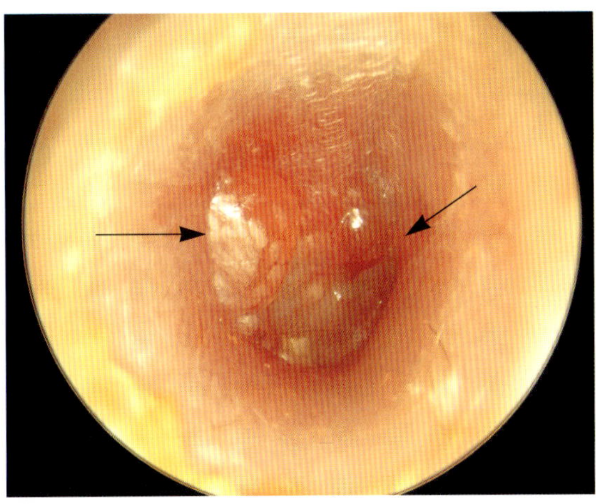

FIGURE 6.16 *Bullous myringitis (right). Bullae on the tympanic membrane (arrowed).*

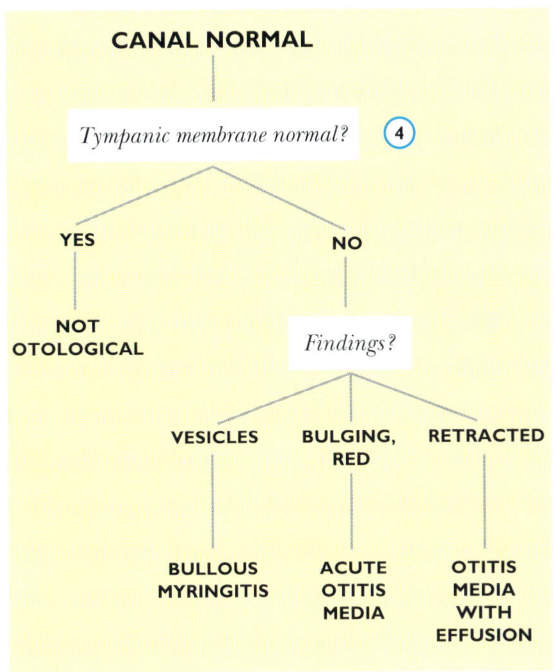

Branch 6.2A

OTITIS MEDIA WITH EFFUSION

As in children, OME is in general a painless condition. However, if it comes on after a sudden change in air pressure (baurotrauma) it can initially be painful. Baurotrauma is discussed in Chapter 8.

NON-OTOLOGIC OTALGIA

If the tympanic membrane is normal, the non-otologic causes of otalgia (Table 6.1) are looked for by examining the area around the ear, the cervical spine, and temporomandibular joint and the mouth and oropharynx. If in doubt about pathology in the latter, specialist referral is important to exclude carcinoma.

CHAPTER 7

THE DISCHARGING EAR

When a patient complains of a discharge from their ear, it is essential to confirm that they are not talking about wax but something that is moist and can be identified as such because it soaks the pillow or requires to be mopped. In many instances such a discharge will have a foul smell. Blood and cerebrospinal fluid (CSF) can also be described as a discharge but these occur most frequently as a result of trauma (Chapter 8).

There are two main conditions that can cause an ear to discharge: otitis externa and active COM. The distinction is made by otoscopy but a history of an associated itch makes otitis externa more likely. On the other hand, a history of previous ear surgery or an associated hearing impairment makes active COM more likely. To confuse the issue, the discharge from active COM may sometimes cause a secondary otitis externa.

Look at summary tree 7.1

When otoscopy is performed on a discharging ear, removal of all pus and debris is essential. This allows the canal skin to be seen and classified as normal or not ①.

OTITIS EXTERNA

Otitis externa is the diagnosis if the canal skin is inflamed (Figure 7.1). In some ears with otitis externa it is not possible to inspect the tympanic membrane because of oedema. With toilet and treatment this should become easier. In others, the tympanic membrane may be seen from the start in which case it may also be affected

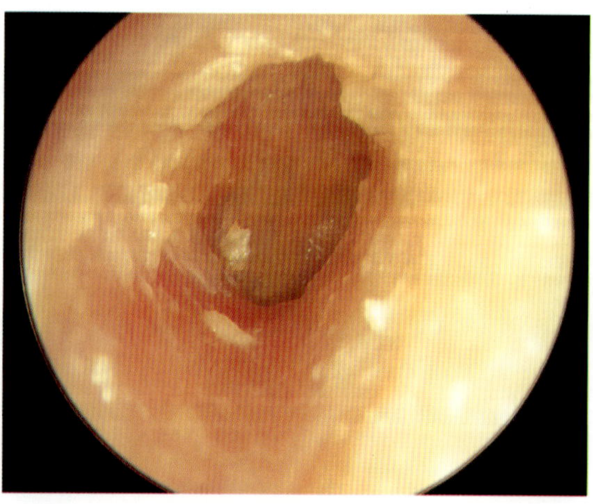

FIGURE 7.1 *Right otitis externa. The discharge is from the underlying oedematous inflamed canal skin.*

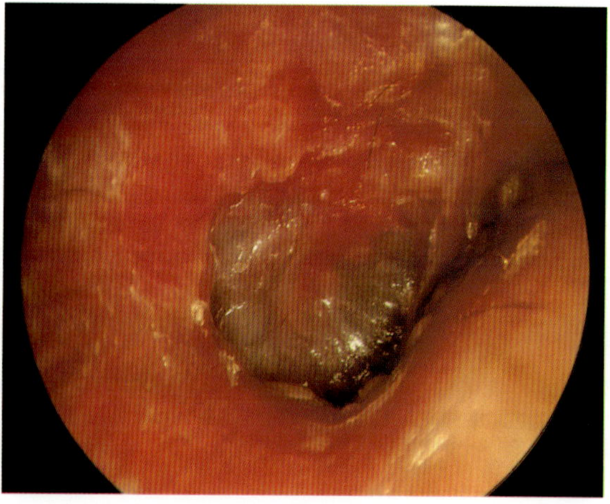

FIGURE 7.2 *Same ear as Figure 7.1 after toilet. The epithelium of the tympanic membrane can be seen to be inflamed.*

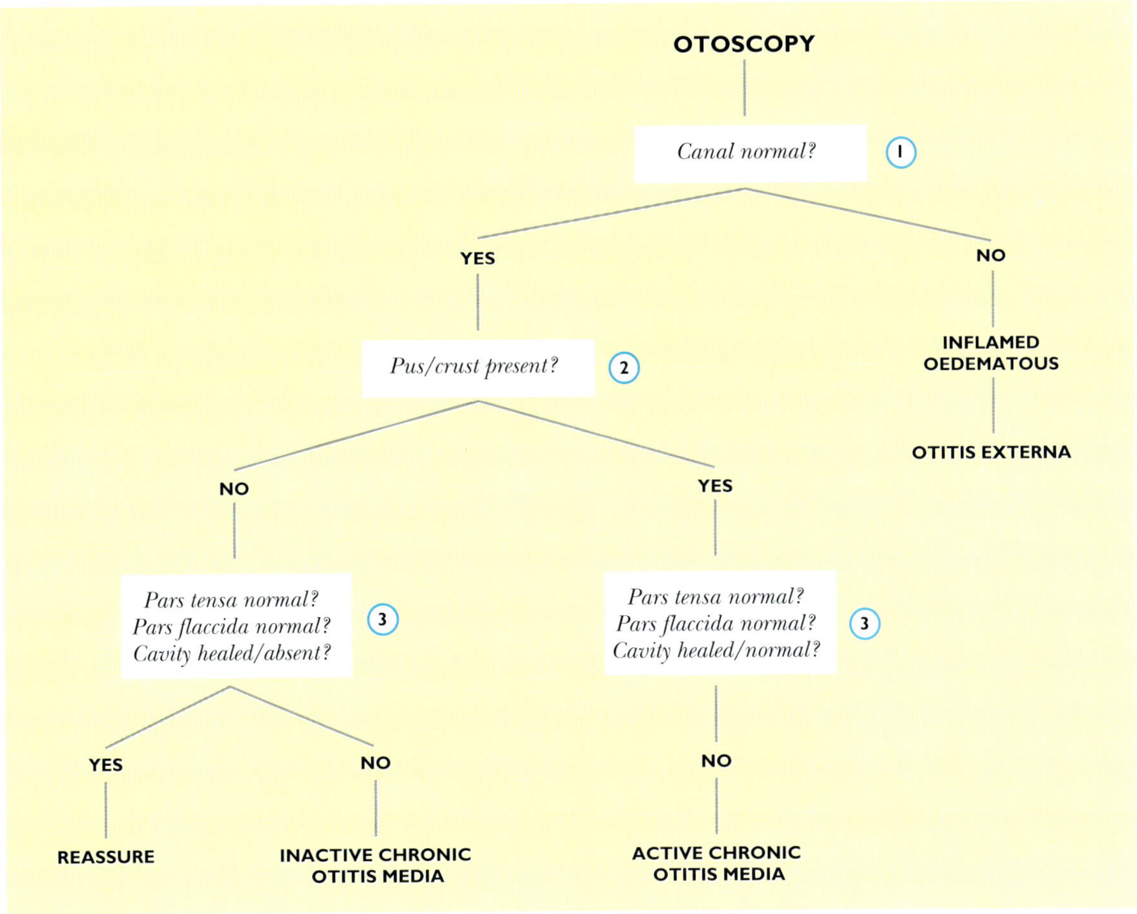

OTOSCOPY

Canal normal? ①

YES — NO

YES

Pus/crust present? ②

NO

INFLAMED OEDEMATOUS

OTITIS EXTERNA

NO — **YES**

Pars tensa normal?
Pars flaccida normal?
Cavity healed/absent? ③

Pars tensa normal?
Pars flaccida normal?
Cavity healed/normal? ③

YES — **NO**

NO

REASSURE

INACTIVE CHRONIC OTITIS MEDIA

ACTIVE CHRONIC OTITIS MEDIA

Summary tree 7.1 Discharging ear.

(Figure 7.2). It is important that the tympanic membrane be assessed at some stage to exclude active chronic otitis media as the cause of the otitis externa.

Management

Otitis externa most frequently presents as an itchy discomfort rather than as a discharge, so its management is discussed elsewhere (see pages 48–49). When monitoring the effect of such treatment, the inexperienced should be wary of interpreting ear drops as an inflammatory discharge (Figure 7.3).

Look at summary tree 7.1

Having excluded otitis externa as a cause of a reported discharge, the tympanic membrane

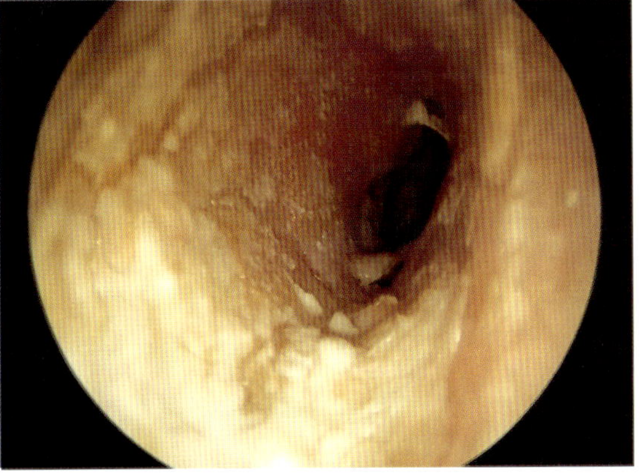

FIGURE 7.3 *Right canal coated with white ear drops (gentamicin hydrocortisone). This can sometimes be mistaken for a discharge.*

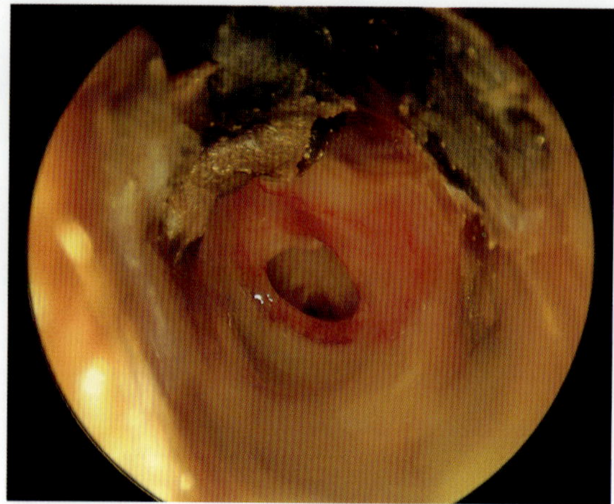

FIGURE 7.4 *Left active chronic otitis media. Pus and dried pus coats the ear canal. There is an anterior pars tensa perforation, through which the middle ear mucosa can be seen to be inflamed.*

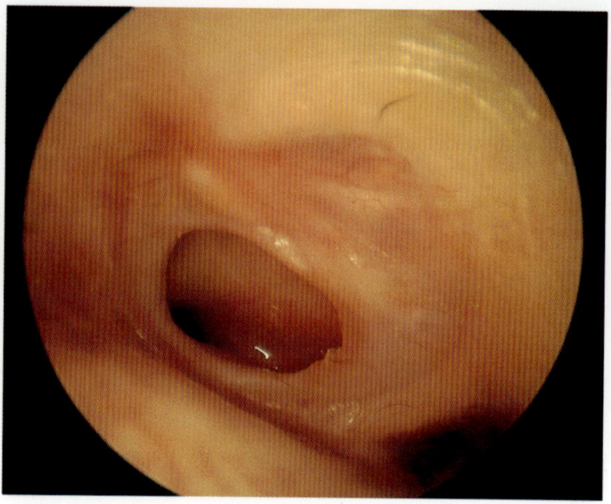

FIGURE 7.5 *Same ear as Figure 7.4 after aural toilet. A clearer view is obtained of the perforation and the inflamed middle ear mucosa.*

should be visible. If pus or debris has not been removed to achieve this, then the next question is whether the ear is currently active as evidenced by pus or crusting ② (Figure 7.4). Crusts are often mistaken for wax rather than dried pus.

ACTIVE CHRONIC OTITIS MEDIA

Crusts imply active COM which will be evident after their removal (Figure 7.5). If the ear is discharging at the time of the examination, it may be difficult to assess despite meticulous cleaning. A red inflamed area is often all that can be seen but the diagnosis is almost certainly active COM. Regular aural toilet over the next few days should allow the ear to settle sufficiently for it to be better assessed.

All patients with active chronic otitis media should have a specialist assessment, because complications are frequent (Table 7.1) and the risks of these can be lessened or avoided by appropriate medical or surgical management. In a specific patient, assessment of the risks and choice of management requires an expert opinion. As this is the case, the non-specialist needs only to decide whether there is active COM or not. This decision is based on the finding of pus or inflammation. Unfortunately,

TABLE 7.1 *Potential complications of active chronic otitis media*

Complications	Symptoms	Pathology
Frequent	Hearing impairment	Ossicular erosion
	Vertigo/imbalance	Labyrinthitis
Less common	Hearing impairment	Cochlear damage
	Facial palsy	VIIth nerve damage
Rare	Headaches, unconsciousness	Intracranial abscess

these are frequently missed because of inexperience in knowing where to look. There are three main areas to assess ③.

Look at summary tree 7.1 ③

Q *Is the pars tensa normal?*

If the chronic otitis media primarily affects the middle ear there will be a permanent defect of the pars tensa. When such an ear is active, the middle ear mucosa as seen through the perforation will be inflamed and producing mucopus (Figure 7.5). This contrasts with the appearance of the mucosa when the ear is inactive (see Chapter 4, and Figure 4.1). The site and size of the perforation varies as does the degree of

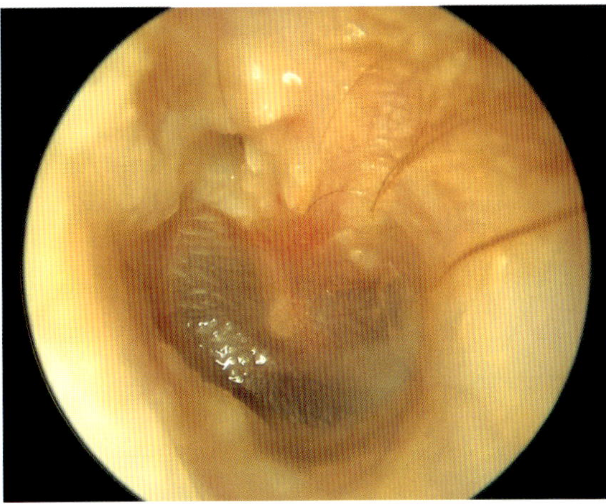

FIGURE 7.6 *Left active chronic otitis media. Pars flaccida obscured by pus. The pars tensa is normal.*

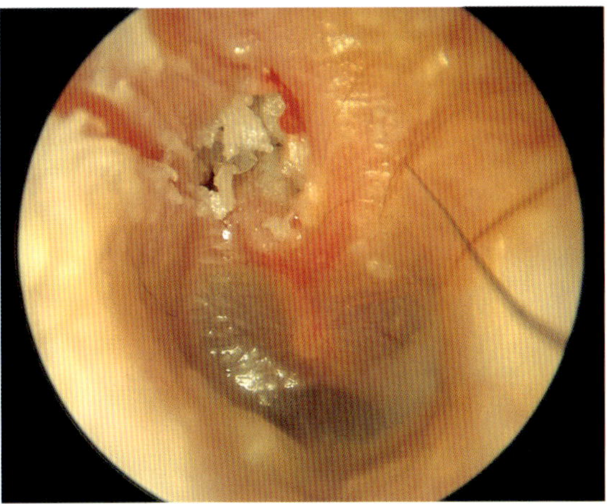

FIGURE 7.7 *Same ear as Figure 7.6 after aural toilet. Active chronic otitis media clearly visible affecting pars flaccida in the attic. The white debris is squamous epithelial debris, indicative of a cholesteatoma.*

mucosal oedema but this is not of any diagnostic or management significance to the non-specialist. Sometimes an aural polyp may (Figure 7.22) or may not (Figure 7.21) obscure the view of the tympanic membrane. Referral of such patients for specialist management should not be delayed because they are more likely to develop complications.

Q Is the pars flaccida normal?

The pars flaccida is one of the areas where active chronic otitis media can be missed. This is because in many instances the diseased area is limited and frequently covered by a dried crust of pus (Figure 7.6). When such crusts are removed, the active COM will become obvious (Figure 7.7).

There are several histological variants of active COM, one of which is a cholesteatoma. This usually starts as a localised retraction pocket of the pars flaccida which retains its epithelial debris and excites an inflammatory reaction around it. Most cholesteatomas present as active COM of the pars flaccida in the attic.

Q If a mastoid cavity is present, is it healed?

Surgery for active COM sometimes results in an open mastoid cavity. These are sometimes missed unless the examiner knows where to look. This can be made more difficult by a narrow external auditory canal which has not been surgically enlarged (meatoplasty) to allow the cavity to be self-cleansing. Mastoid cavities are created to enable more thorough removal of disease in the attic and antrum. This is achieved by removing the posterosuperior canal wall and opening up the mastoid air cell system (Figure 7.8). The aim is to have a cavity lined by self-cleansing skin and it appears as a dry, postero-superior enlargement of the canal. These can easily be missed when the ear is examined via a speculum (Figures 7.9 and 7.10).

Unfortunately some mastoid cavities do not heal and continue to discharge. This possibility should be considered, therefore, in someone with an ear discharge who has had surgery. The appearances of active cavities are varied, but most frequently there is pus (Figure 7.11) which when removed reveals an inflamed mucosa (Figure 7.12). As in pars flaccida disease, the inexperienced should be aware that what looks like wax in the posterosuperior canal wall can indeed be a large plug of dried pus that fills and hides a mastoid cavity (Figure 7.13). Needless to say, the pars tensa should also be assessed when

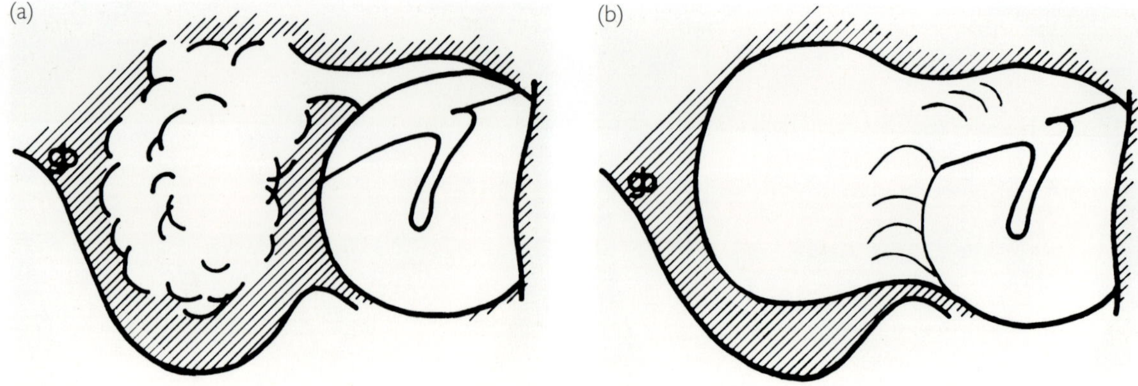

FIGURE 7.8 *(a) Diagram of normal right ear and mastoid air cell system. (b) Right modified radical mastoidectomy created by removing posterior canal wall to connect mastoid air cells with the canal.*

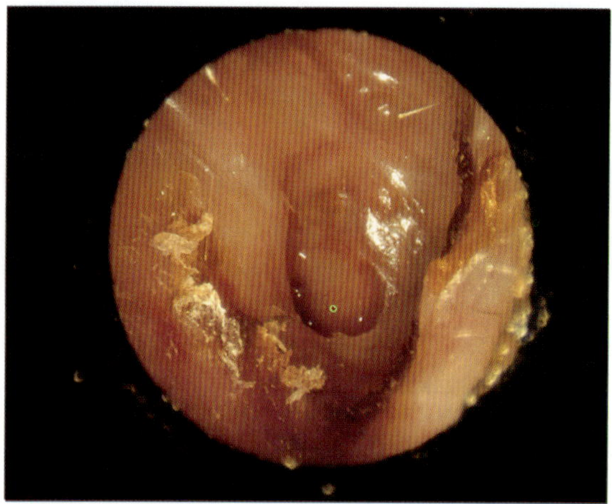

FIGURE 7.9 *Right ear. Limited view of posterosuperior canal wall because of angle of vision and a small speculum.*

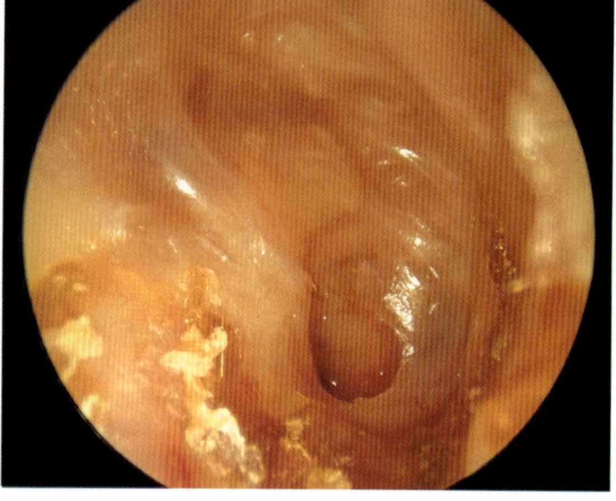

FIGURE 7.10 *Right modified radical mastoidectomy. Same ear as Figure 7.9 with wider angle of view. The presence posterosuperiorly of an open mastoid cavity is now obvious. In this ear the cavity is healed but there is a perforation of the pars tensa through which the middle ear mucosa is seen to be inflamed and is the site of activity.*

there is a cavity because it is frequently perforated (Figures 7.10 and 7.12) and there may or may not be active middle ear disease in addition.

Management

Whilst the patient is awaiting a specialist opinion aural toilet should be instituted. This can include syringing (see page 83) even if an open mastoid cavity is present. The patient can also be instructed in how to self-mop their ear with cotton buds (see page 84). If the specialist subsequently decides against surgical intervention, the patient is frequently referred back to the primary care physician for management. As well as aural toilet this may include topical steroid/antibiotic ear drops or sprays.

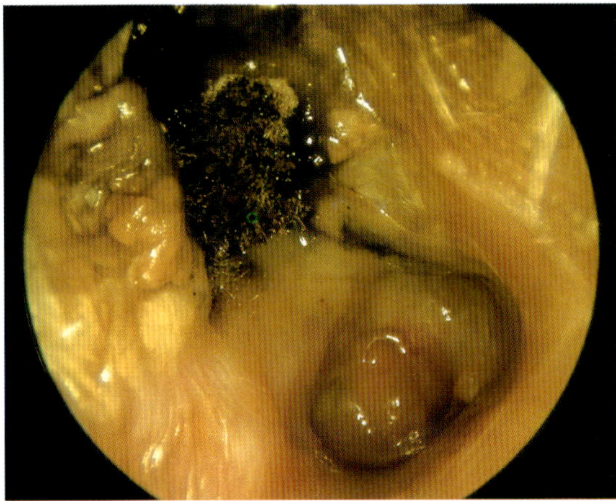

FIGURE 7.11 *Right active chronic otitis media in an open mastoid cavity. The mastoid cavity is active with pus and dried crusts.*

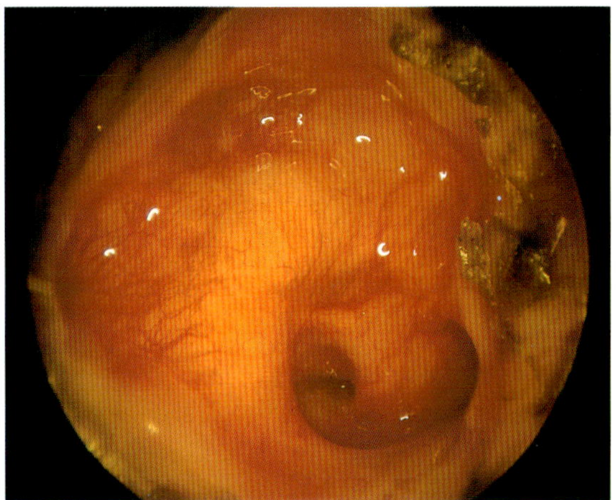

FIGURE 7.12 *Same ear as Figure 7.11 after aural toilet. The lining of the mastoid cavity is grossly inflamed and in parts there is granulation tissue. In addition the middle ear is inflamed as seen through a subtotal pars tensa perforation.*

SPECIALIST – LOOK AT SUMMARY TREE 7.2

The specialist Summary tree is different from Summary tree 7.1 in that it breaks down active chronic otitis into active mucosal and active squamous disease, an important distinction for specialists to make.

ACTIVE CHRONIC OTITIS MEDIA – SPECIALIST

The specialist has several objectives when a patient is referred with active COM. The first objective is to define the areas involved and the type of disease. This is done after aural toilet usually with the aid of an operating microscope. If the ear is particularly active, then aural toilet may have to be repeated over several days or weeks to allow the ear to settle sufficiently for it to be assessed. The anatomical area or areas affected will be any combination of middle ear, attic and mastoid cavity. The type of activity in each will be defined as being mucosal or squamous epithelial disease.

The second objective is to decide how to alleviate the patient's symptoms of discharge and any associated hearing impairment. In suitably trained hands, this is best achieved

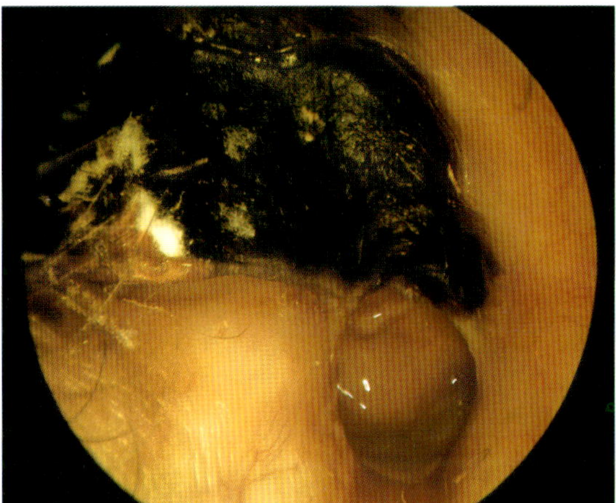

FIGURE 7.13 *Right active chronic otitis media. There is a large crust on the posterosuperior canal wall. The pars tensa is perforated and there is active mucosal disease which could be thought to be the sole cause of the ear discharge. The crust fills and hides an active mastoid cavity.*

permanently by surgery irrespective of the site or type of disease. When there is active mucosal disease, medical management is an alternative option but this is not the case when there is

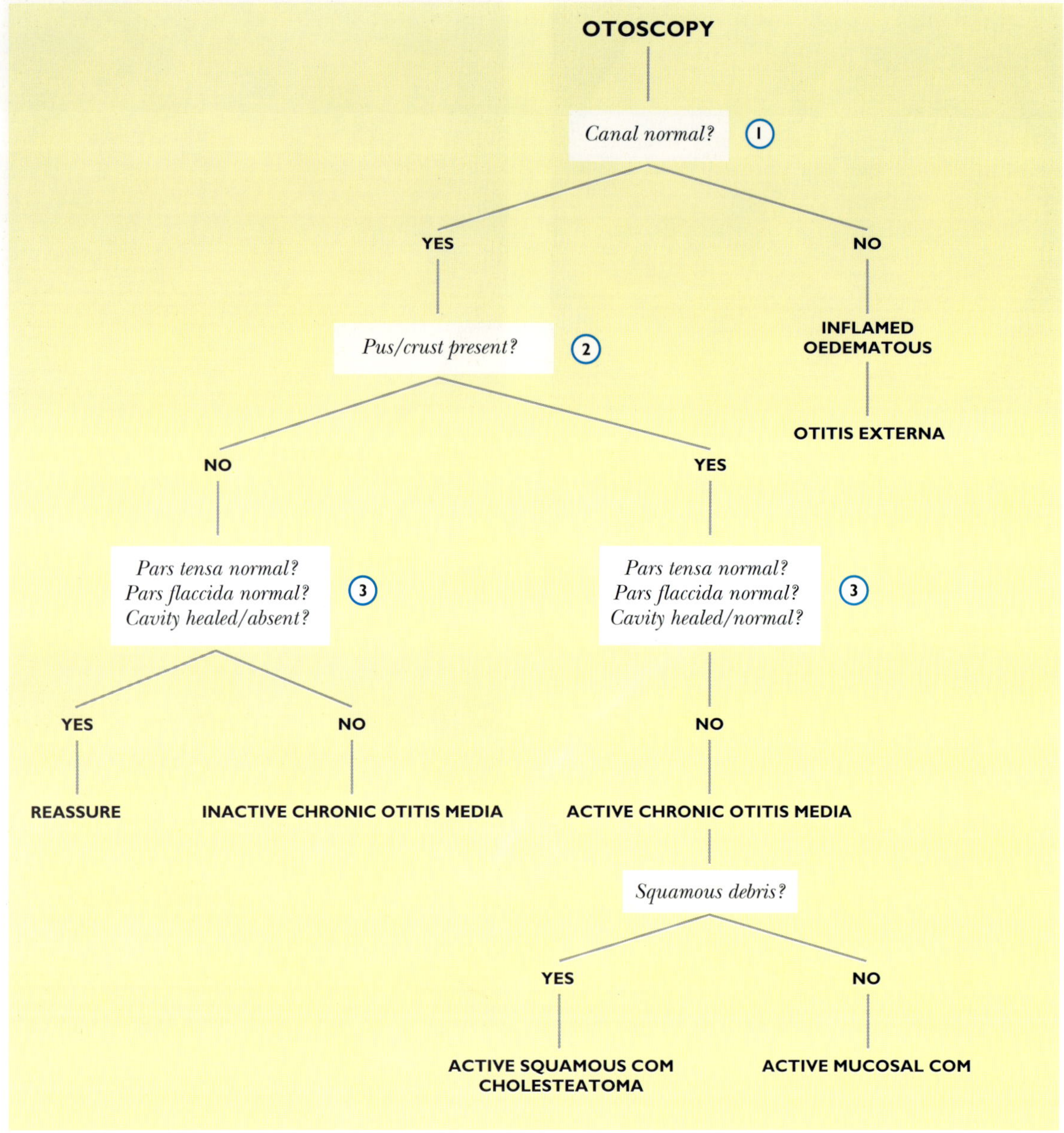

Summary tree 7.2 Discharging ear – specialist.

active squamous disease. Irrespective of the types of disease a hearing aid is an option to consider to alleviate any hearing disability, although the earmould of the aid may exacerbate a discharge.

The third objective is to prevent complications (Table 7.1). Again, this is best achieved by making the ear permanently inactive. This is most reliably achieved by surgery, although surgery itself can sometimes cause the same complications. Some consider that active squamous disease is more frequently associated with complications and, correspondingly, should be more aggressively treated. However,

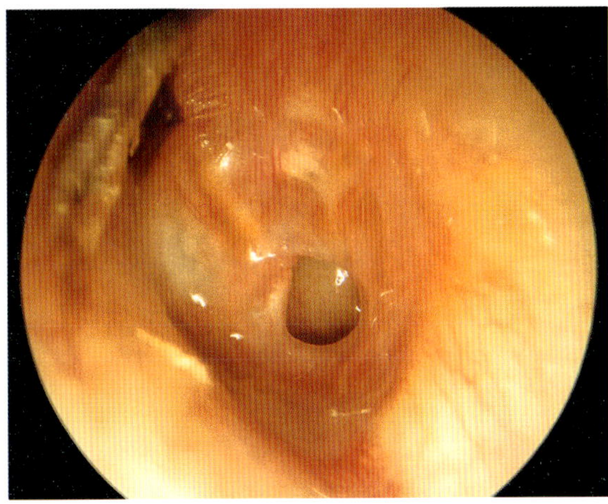

FIGURE 7.14 *Left active mucosal chronic otitis media. There is pus in the canal which comes through a 20% posterior pars tensa perforation from a moderately inflamed middle ear mucosa.*

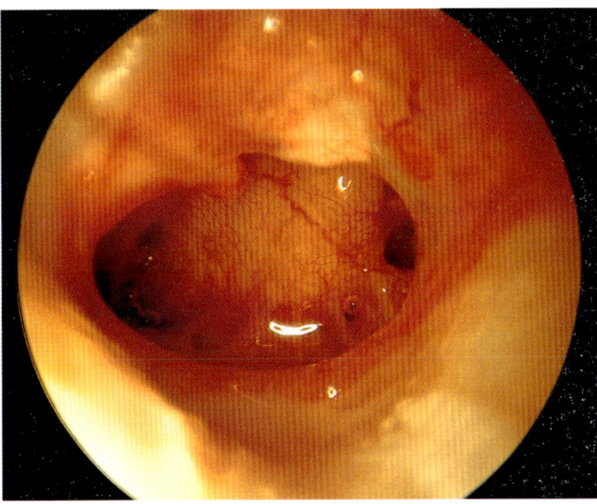

FIGURE 7.15 *Left active mucosal chronic otitis media. There is pus on the canal wall. The middle ear mucosa, seen through a 60% inferior pars tensa perforation, is hyperaemic but not grossly oedematous.*

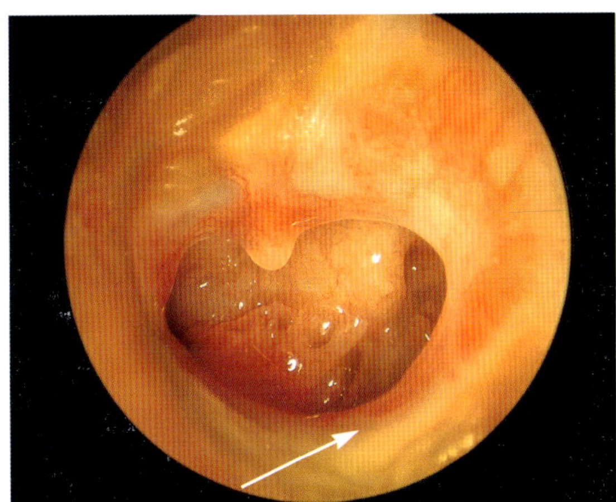

FIGURE 7.16 *Left active mucosal chronic otitis media. There is pus on the canal wall. The middle ear mucosa, seen through a 60% inferior pars tensa perforation, is minimally inflamed. The activity is mainly from granulation tissue on the edge of the perforation (arrowed).*

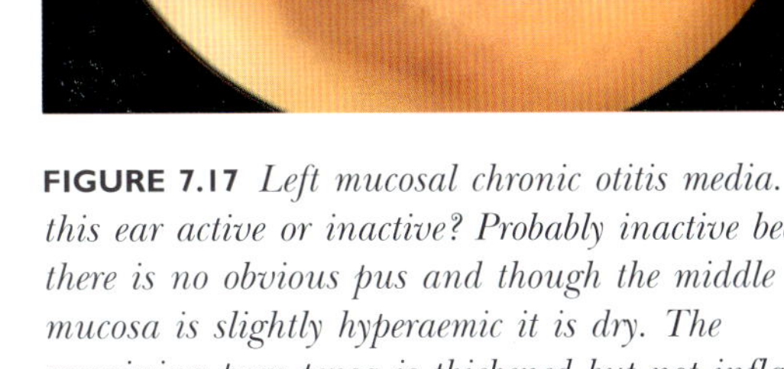

FIGURE 7.17 *Left mucosal chronic otitis media. Is this ear active or inactive? Probably inactive because there is no obvious pus and though the middle ear mucosa is slightly hyperaemic it is dry. The remaining pars tensa is thickened but not inflamed.*

the greater 'unsafeness' of active squamous disease has yet to be proven.

Assessment

Active COM has many different appearances depending on what area is affected and the type of disease. Surgery, and in particular the creation of an open mastoid cavity, can complicate the picture. Thus it is impossible to illustrate all the possibilities, but hopefully by giving examples categorised by anatomical site, the principles of assessment can be learned.

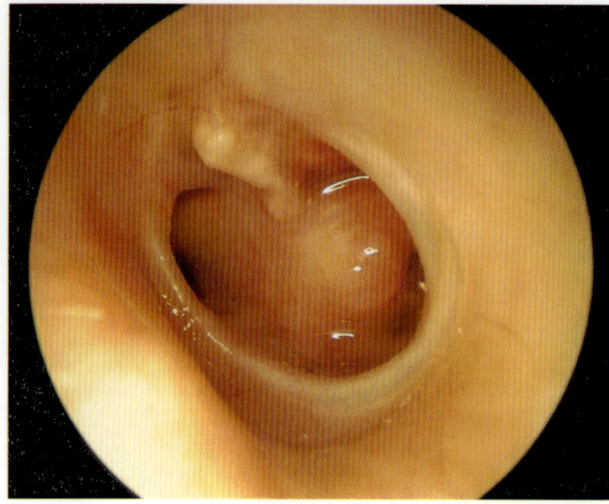

FIGURE 7.18 *Left mucosal chronic otitis media. Is this ear active or inactive? Probably active because the middle ear mucosa seen through an 80% perforation is oedematous and wet with mucus. There is an area of slight mucosal hypertrophy posteriorly in the middle ear.*

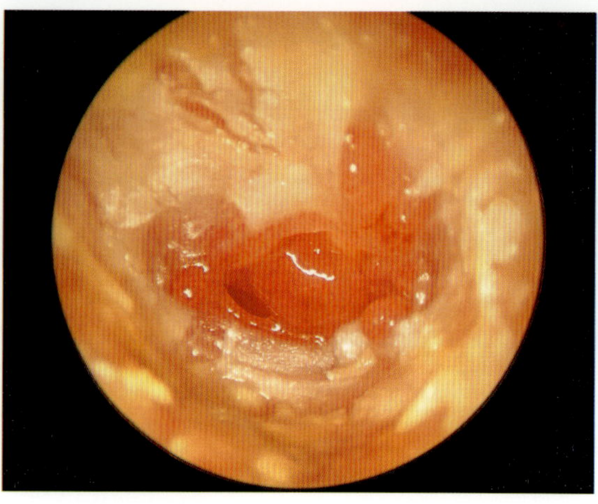

FIGURE 7.19 *Left active mucosal chronic otitis media. There is pus and debris on the canal wall. The tympanic membrane cannot be fully visualised but there appears to be an inferior defect. The main finding is a polyp protruding through the perforation and granulation tissue on the remaining tympanic membrane.*

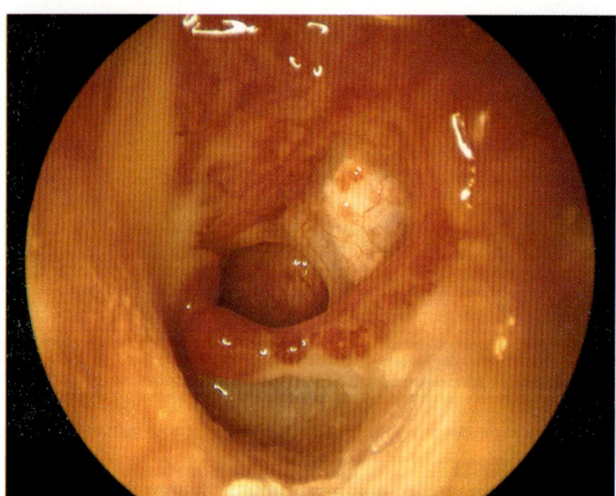

FIGURE 7.20 *Left active mucosal chronic otitis media. The activity in this ear is primarily of granulation tissue on the pars tensa and pars flaccida. The 20% anterior pars tensa perforation and middle ear mucosa disease is less relevant.*

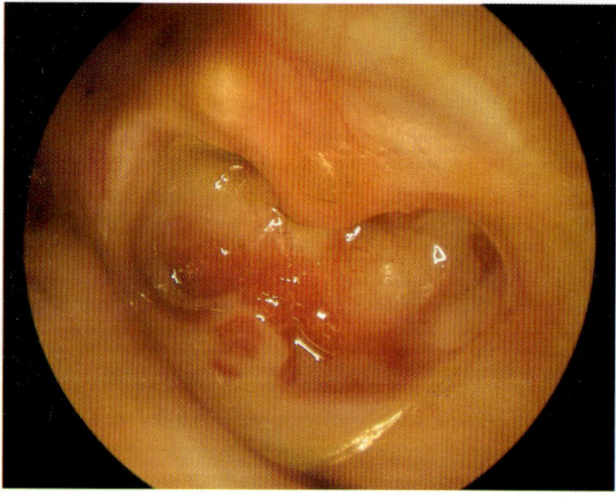

FIGURE 7.21 *Left active mucosal chronic otitis media. There is a collection of pus inferiorly arising primarily from gross granulations in the inferior middle ear (hypotympanum). There is a 60% inferior pars tensa perforation.*

Pars tensa: mucosal disease (Figures 7.14 to 7.23)

If active COM affects the pars tensa it is most commonly mucosal disease. The degree of mucosal inflammation varies from mild oedema to exuberant granulation tissue and polyps (Figures 7.14 to 7.23). How much of the middle ear mucosa can be seen is determined by the

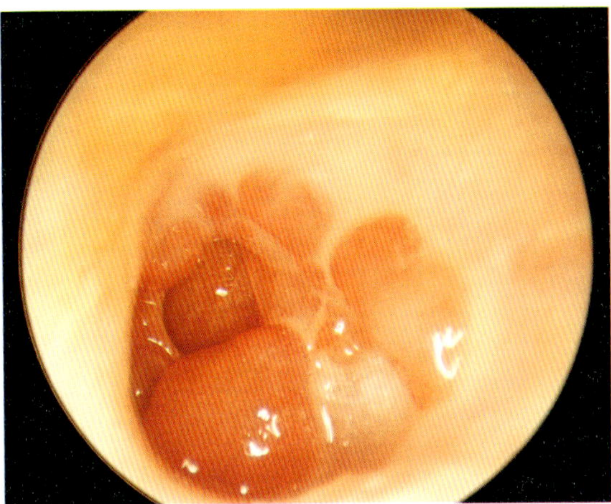

FIGURE 7.22 *Left active mucosal chronic otitis media. There is pus in the canal and an inferior polyp. There appears to be a 20% anterior pars tensa perforation but anatomical landmarks such as the handle of the malleus are not obvious because of oedema and scars.*

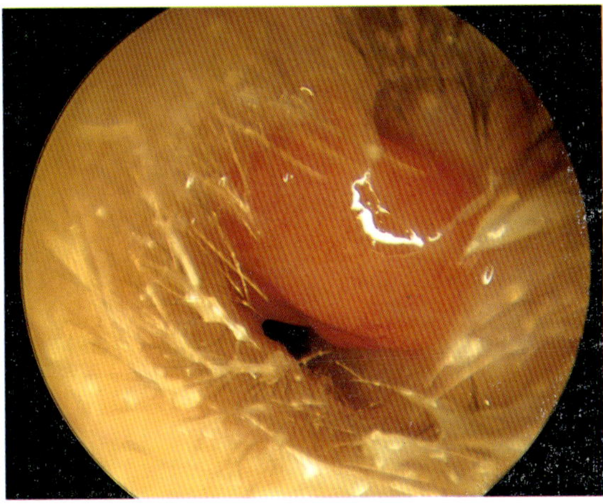

FIGURE 7.23 *Left active chronic otitis media. The canal is visually obstructed by a large polyp but the ear is obviously active due to chronic otitis media. This polyp could arise from middle ear or attic disease but it requires to be removed to make the distinction.*

size of the pars tensa defect and whether the view is obstructed by polyps. Not infrequently the ossicular chain is eroded by the mucosal inflammation, the long process of the incus being at particular risk (see Figure 3.12 page 15 and Figure 4.13 page 22). The stapes super-structure (see Figure 4.16 page 22) and the handle of the malleus (see Figure 4.17 page 23) can also be eroded. Sometimes the activity is mainly from granulation tissue around the edges of the perforation rather than from the middle ear. If there are granulations on an apparently intact pars tensa, the much less frequent diagnosis of granular myringitis has to be considered (see page 73). Finally if the activity is primarily posterior, there may be active squamous disease in a posterior retraction pocket (see below).

Management

Topical antibiotic and steroid drops, when given in addition to aural toilet, are of proven value in the management of active mucosal disease. Unfortunately, the chances of the activity recurring are high. As some of the antibiotics in proprietary antibiotic steroid drops are potentially ototoxic, care ought to be exercised

in their continued use, especially if the ear becomes inactive. The preferred option for long-term management is surgery.

The surgical management of active mucosal disease is to graft the tympanic membrane defect (myringoplasty) and this is technically easier to do if an active ear is first made inactive. Should aural toilet and topical antibiotic steroid drops not achieve this, surgery should still be performed. Some advocate a cortical mastoidec-tomy in addition to a myringoplasty, but it is more relevant to ensure free drainage past any residual ossicular chain by removing granula-tion tissue and taking out the incus if its long process has been eroded.

Pars tensa – squamous disease (middle ear cholesteatoma) (Figures 7.24 to 7.26)

Middle ear retraction pockets, particularly if they affect the posterosuperior quadrant, can sometimes progress to active squamous epithe-lial disease – a cholesteatoma. Why this occurs is unclear but it is generally held that when the retraction is no longer self-cleansing, retention of epithelial debris occurs which excites an inflammatory response. Hence, the earliest sign

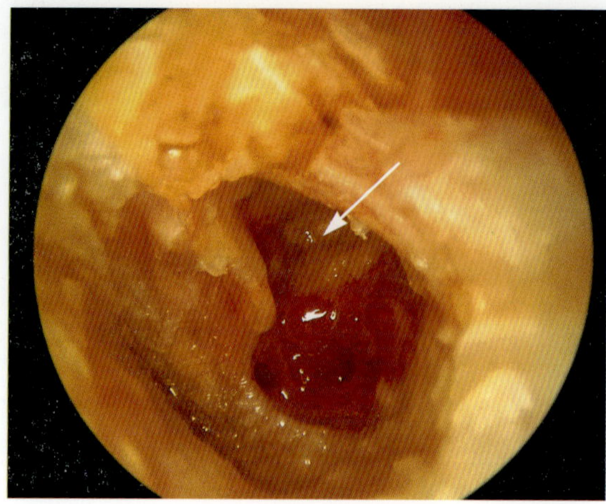

FIGURE 7.24 *Left active squamous chronic otitis media. There is pus and squamous debris in the canal and a posterior retraction of the pars tensa (arrowed). Within the retraction pocket there are granulations.*

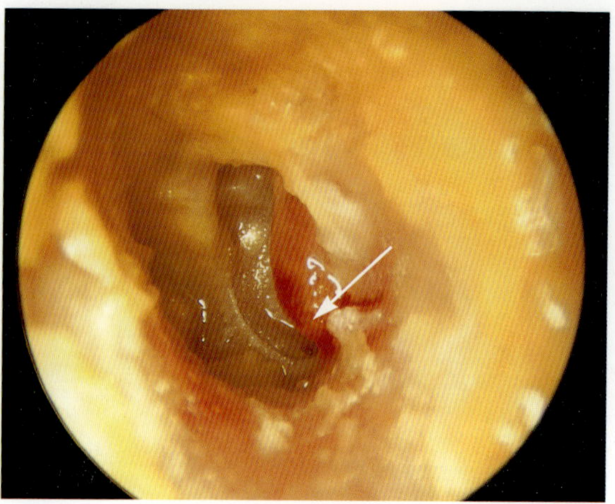

FIGURE 7.25 *Left active squamous chronic otitis media. There is pus and squamous debris in the canal and a posterior retraction of the pars tensa. There is granulation tissue on the posterior canal wall (arrowed) presumably excited by retained epithelial debris in the retraction pocket which is out of view.*

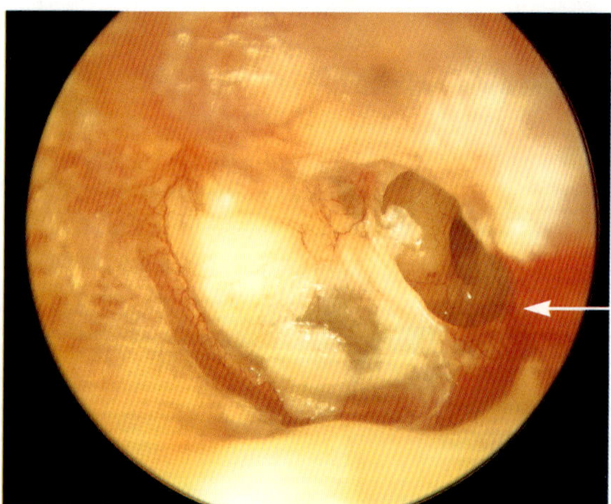

FIGURE 7.26 *Left active chronic otitis media. There is pus in the external auditory canal and granulations on the posterior canal wall (arrowed). The appearance is similar but not identical to Figure 7.25 in that the pars tensa is perforated rather than retracted. There may or may not be retained epithelial debris out of vision.*

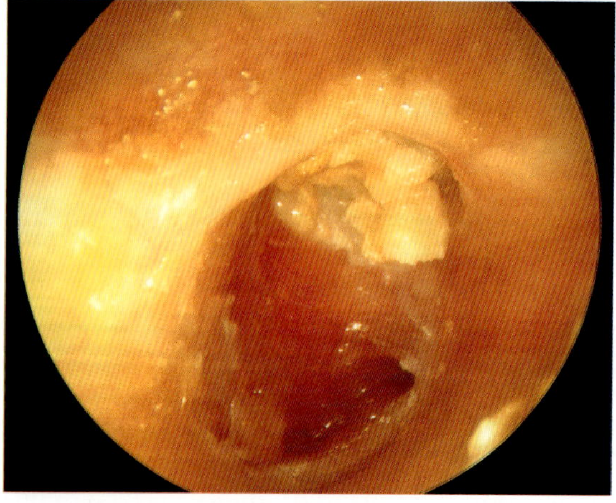

FIGURE 7.27 *Right active squamous chronic otitis media. There is pus and debris in the canal. In the attic there is obvious white keratinous debris indicative of a cholesteatoma of the pars flaccida. The pars tensa is probably intact but inflamed.*

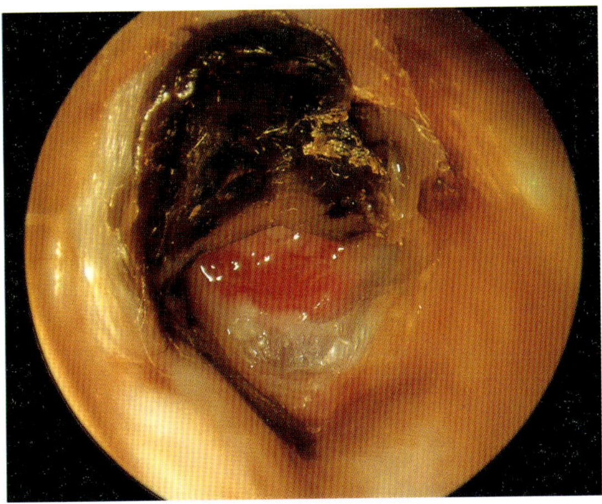

FIGURE 7.28 *Right active squamous chronic otitis media. There is pus in the canal and a crust of dried pus in the attic. There are granulations on the pars tensa but if the attic crust were removed an attic cholesteatoma would be evident (see Figure 7.29).*

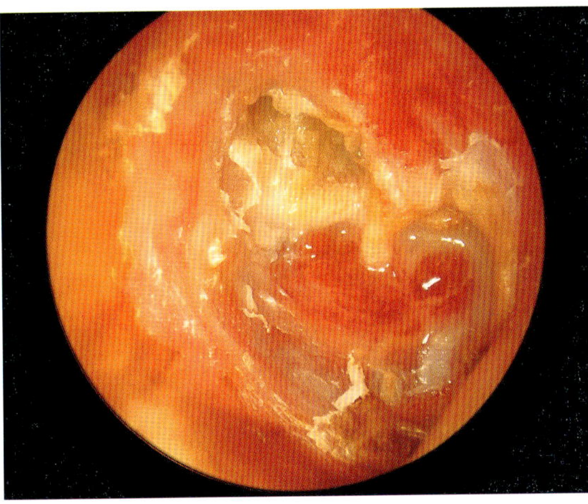

FIGURE 7.29 *Same ear as Figure 7.28 after removal of pus and crusts. The granulations on the pars tensa remain but in addition a retraction of the pars flaccida is evident with retained epithelial debris.*

of a cholesteatoma occurring in a middle ear retraction pocket is often the appearance of granulations on the posterior canal wall. The extent to which the white retained epithelium within the retraction pocket is evident can vary.

Management
The principles of management of cholesteatoma in the middle ear are the same as in attic disease. They are therefore discussed together (see below).

Pars flaccida – squamous disease (attic cholesteatoma) (Figures 7.28 to 7.33)

The most frequent type of COM to affect the pars flaccida is squamous disease. Simple retractions of the pars flaccida are common (Figure 7.31) but sometimes these become active because they are not self-cleansing of squamous epithelial debris (Figure 7.32).

The clinical detection of attic disease often depends on the removal of an attic crust (Figures 7.28–7.30). The presence of white squamous debris is diagnostic of active squamous disease (cholesteatoma) (Figures 7.27 and 7.29) though sometimes it is less obvious (Figure 7.32).

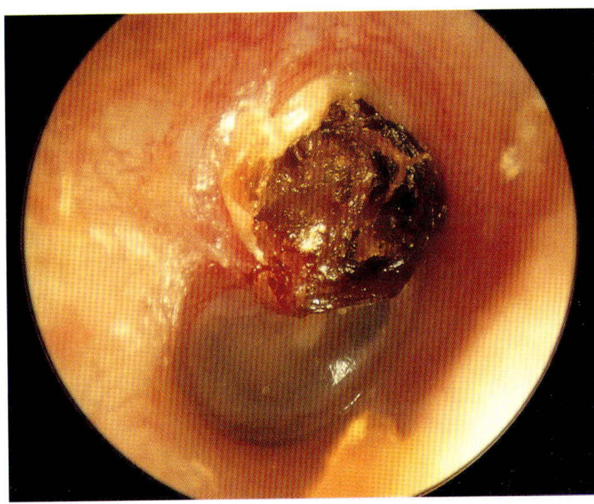

FIGURE 7.30 *Right active squamous chronic otitis media. As there is no pus in the canal and the pars tensa is normal, this ear might be considered normal. The crust in the attic is not wax but dried pus which if removed would reveal an attic cholesteatoma similar to Figure 7.27.*

Management of squamous disease (cholesteatoma) in the middle ear and attic
The simplest procedure for active squamous disease is suction but there is always part of the

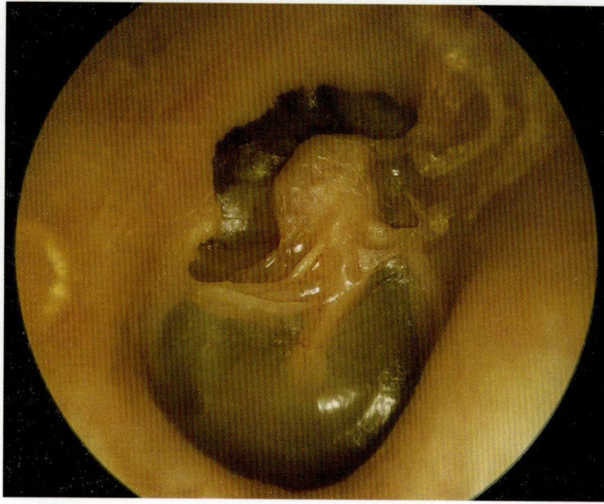

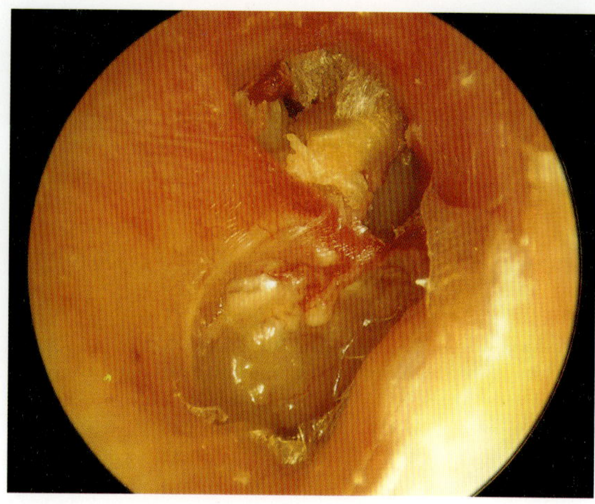

FIGURES 7.31 and 7.32 *These figures should be considered together. In Figure 7.31 (on the left) there is a large pars flaccida retraction in the right attic. Though part of the retraction is out of vision and the bony canal wall has at some time been eroded to expose the head of the malleus and body of the incus, there is no evidence of activity. There is no epithelial debris in the retraction pocket which is presumably self-cleansing. The diagnosis is inactive (squamous) chronic otitis media. In Figure 7.32 (on the right) the anatomy is similar to Figure 7.31 but there is obvious activity. There is pus in the canal, and the skin of the superior canal adjacent to the attic bony erosion is inflamed. There is debris within the retracted pars flaccida. The diagnosis is active squamous chronic otitis media, or cholesteatoma.*

epithelial retraction pocket that cannot be visualised and cleaned out. Thus, surgical exposure of the entire sac is considered advisable and best achieved initially by atticotomy. If this does not expose the epithelial sac, the atticotomy is extended posterior to the ossicles into the mastoid antrum, creating an attico-antrostomy. Cholesteatoma sacs larger than that require the posterior canal wall to be lowered to create a modified radical mastoidectomy. The size of the cavity depends on the degree of sclerosis there has been of the mastoid air cell system. A radical cavity is where all remnants of the ossicular chain and tympanic membrane are removed; this is now seldom the operation of choice because of the desire to surgically improve the hearing and to create a closed middle ear space. Many other approaches have been suggested, the most common being to start from the mastoid air cells and work forward before lowering the posterior canal wall to create a modified radical mastoidectomy. A less frequent technique today is a combined approach (transcanal and transmastoid) to

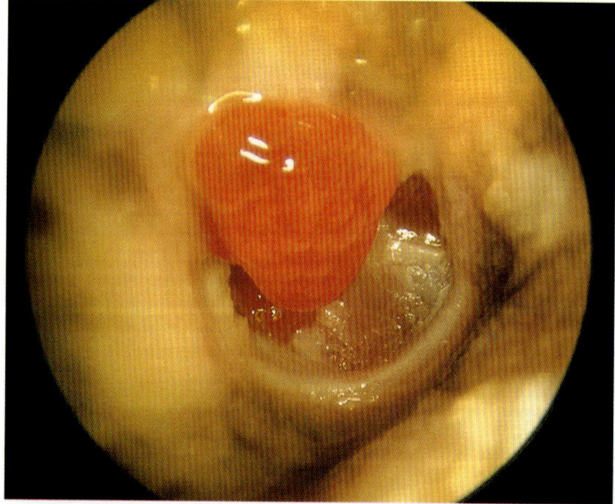

FIGURE 7.33 *Right active chronic otitis media. There is an obvious polyp which appears to originate from the attic. If this is the case, there is almost certainly a cholesteatoma in addition.*

clear out disease with preservation of the posterior canal wall which avoids having an open cavity.

FIGURES 7.34 to 7.38 *Photographs and line drawings of a range of open left sided mastoid cavities selected to illustrate how they can progressively vary in size depending on the extent of the disease and the degree of mastoid pneumatisation. They are all healed and inactive, though some have more debris in them than others. The pars tensa is intact in all except in Figure 7.36.*

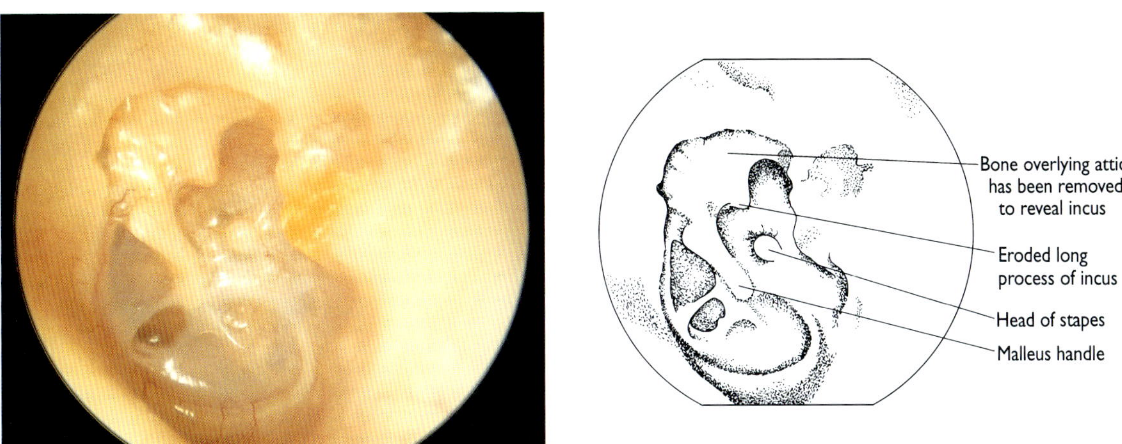

FIGURE 7.34 *Left atticotomy. The attic has been exposed by drilling and is lined by a dry retraction pocket, part of which is out of vision. The malleus handle and body are present, as is the body of the incus. The long process of the incus has been eroded. The pars tensa is intact but retracted onto the head of the stapes.*

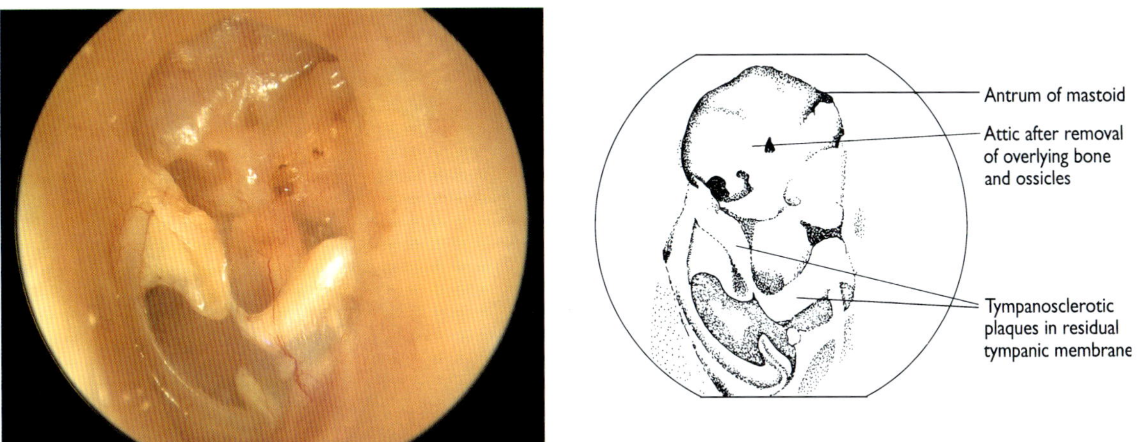

FIGURE 7.35 *Left atticotomy. More of the attic bone has been removed than in Figure 7.34. The ossicles are absent and there are tympanosclerotic plaques in the residual pars tensa.*

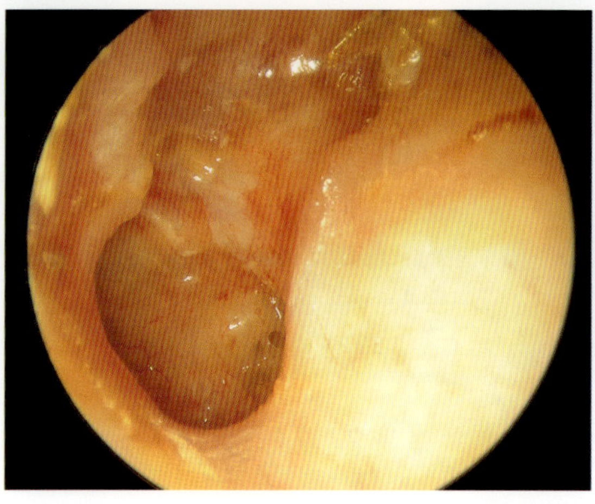
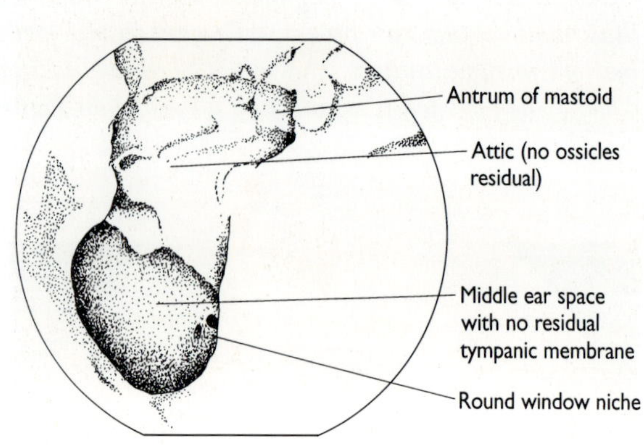

FIGURE 7.36 *Left attico-antrostomy. Both the attic and the antrum have been surgically opened. No ossicles remain and the pars tensa is totally perforated. The middle ear mucosa is inactive and the lining of the attico-antrostomy is dry.*

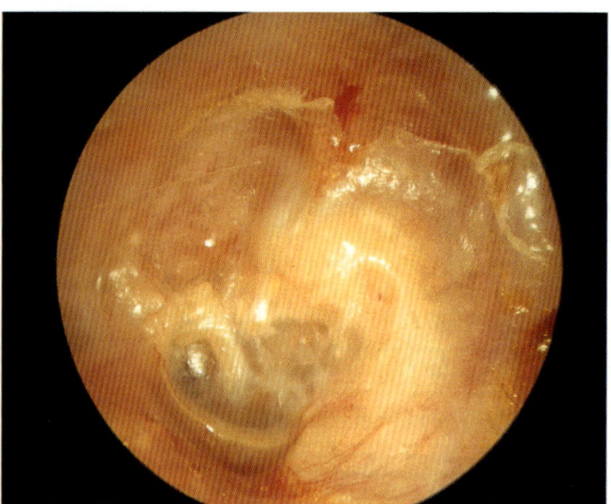
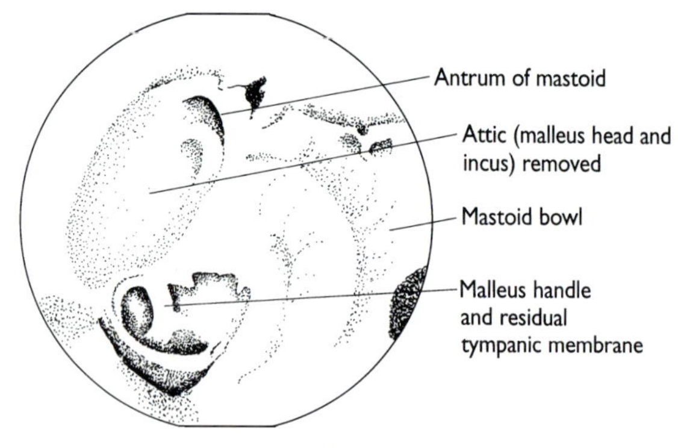

FIGURE 7.37 *Left modified radical mastoidectomy. The mastoid air cells have been opened and the posterior canal wall lowered considerably. The open mastoid cavity is clean and dry. The pars tensa is intact. The handle of the malleus is the only part of the ossicular chain that remains.*

Mastoid cavity disease – general

Figures 7.34 to 7.38 are a series of photographs and line drawings to illustrate the differing extent to which the attic, antrum and mastoid air cells can be opened to expose and remove disease. In Figures 7.34 and 7.35, only the attic has been exposed – an atticotomy. In Figure 7.36 the antrum has been exposed in addition to the attic – an attico-antrostomy. In Figures 7.37 and 7.38 the mastoid air cells have been cleared out and the posterior canal wall lowered down as far as possible without damaging the facial nerve. This creates a healed cavity which

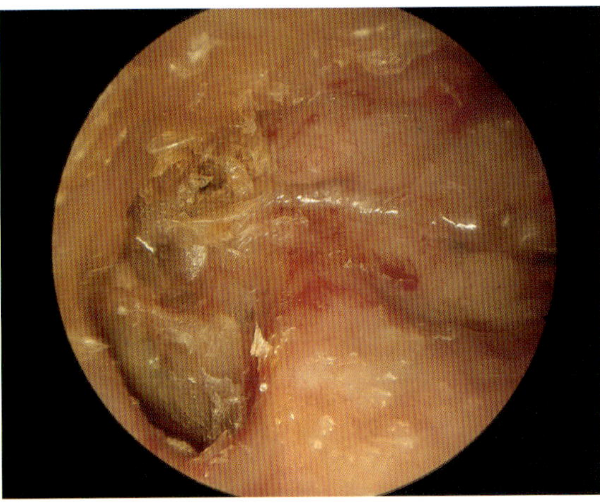

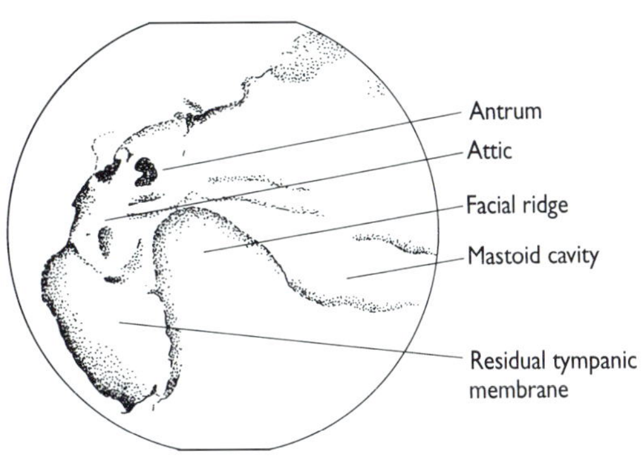

FIGURE 7.38 *Left modified radical mastoidectomy. The open mastoid cavity in this ear is larger than in Figure 7.37. There is crusting in the cavity which would require to be removed to assess the activity. The pars tensa is intact.*

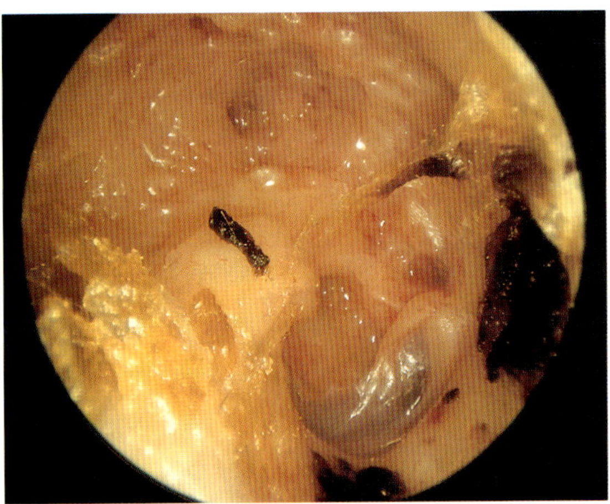

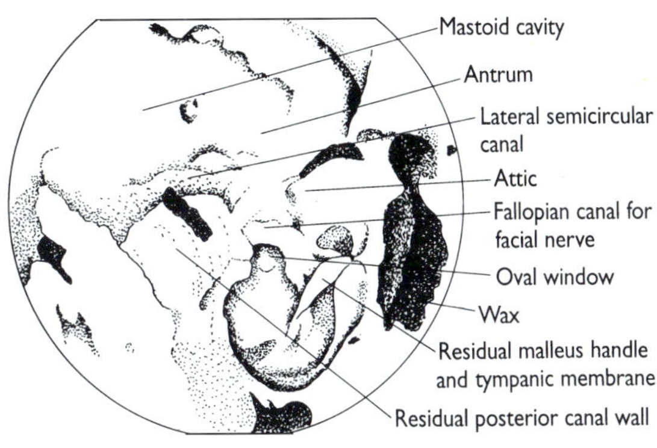

FIGURE 7.39 *Right inactive modified radical mastoidectomy. In the middle ear the handle of the malleus is the only part of the ossicular chain remaining. Anteriorly the pars tensa is retracted but intact creating a small, aerated middle ear space (cava minor). Posteriorly it is retracted and adherent to the promontory. This makes the oval window particularly obvious. The mastoid cavity is healed and inactive. The lateral semicircular canal is prominent in the cavity. The posterior canal wall has not been totally lowered.*

does not retain squamous debris. In this series of photographs, the ears are all inactive both in the middle ear and the cavity. Unfortunately this is not always the case.

Mastoid cavities vary considerably in their appearance. This is because of a combination of factors: the extent of the initial disease, the skill of the surgeon, what reconstruction has been attempted and whether the ear has healed or remains active. If it remains active this may be because of residual disease in the middle ear or mastoid or both and the residual disease may be mucosal, squamous epithelial or both. Figures 7.39 to 7.43 illustrate the various anatomical differences

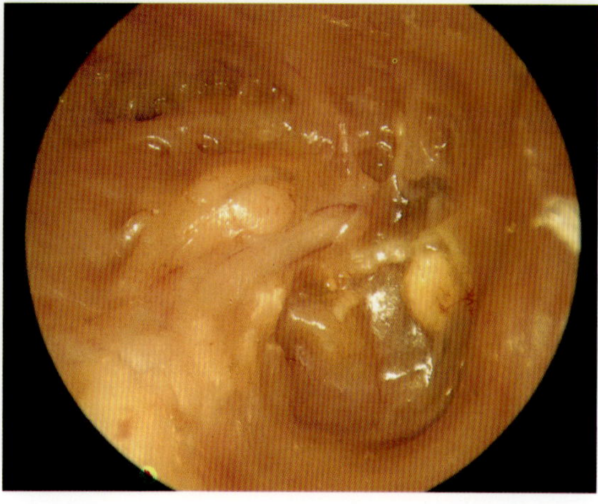

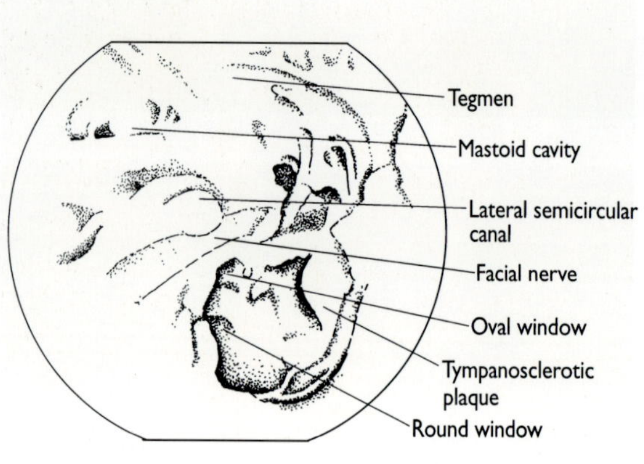

FIGURE 7.40 *Right inactive modified radical mastoidectomy. None of the ossicular chain remains. The oval and round windows are clearly visible posterior to the promontory. There is a retracted membrane over the posterior middle ear but anteriorly there is an aerated middle ear space (cava minor). There is a plaque of tympanosclerosis in the residual pars tensa. The facial nerve has been exposed in its horizontal and initial vertical parts. The mastoid cavity is large with several areas of retraction of its lining into air cells. There is no evidence of activity in the middle ear or mastoid cavity.*

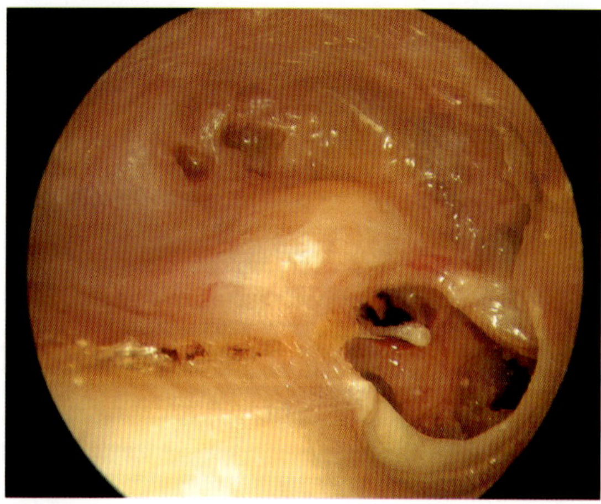

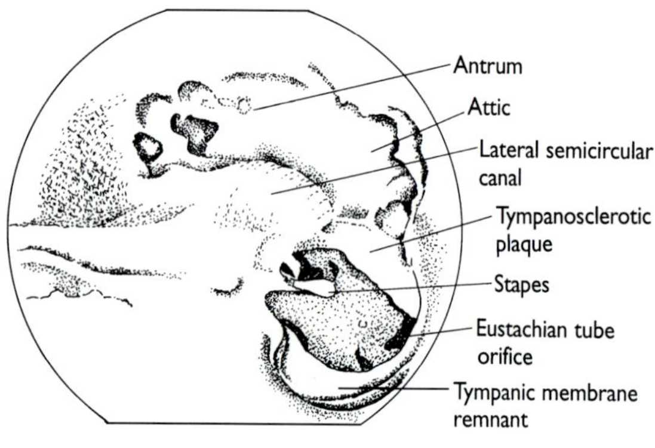

FIGURE 7.41 *Right inactive modified radical mastoidectomy. There is a subtotal perforation of the pars tensa, the anterior remaining part having a tympanosclerotic plaque. The middle ear is inactive. The stapes is the sole remaining ossicle. Its tendon is obvious. Anteriorly the Eustachian tube opening can be seen. There is a large inactive mastoid cavity.*

there can be between cavities. These ears are in the main inactive. Figures 7.44 to 7.49 illustrate various ears with an open mastoid cavity that are active. In some (Figures 7.44 to 7.46) this is solely because of mucosal disease and in others (Figures 7.47 and 7.48) because of residual squamous disease. Invariably in some ears, there is doubt about the type of disease (Figure 7.49). In others, because of reconstructive surgery, recurrent disease and in particular squamous epithelial disease do not

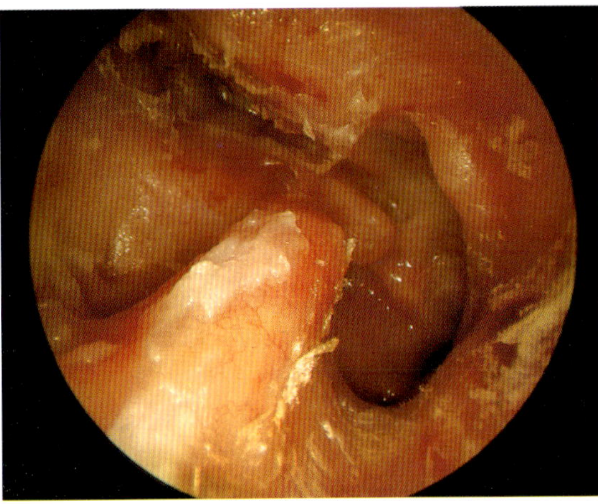

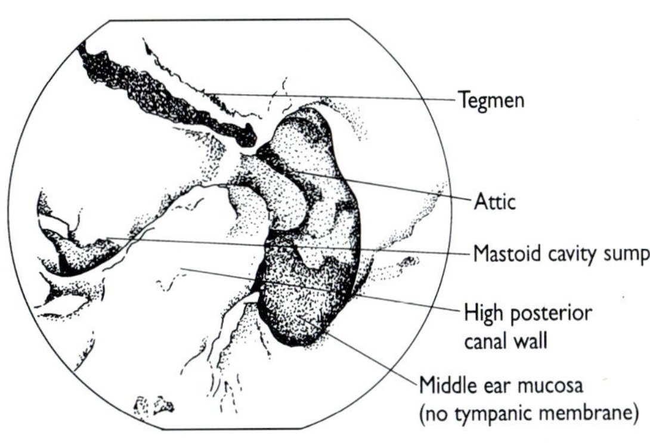

FIGURE 7.42 *Right active modified radical mastoidectomy. There is no residual pars tensa or ossicular chain. The middle ear mucosa is active. The posterior canal wall has not been lowered below the attic. This creates a mastoid bowl with a sump. Part of the lining of the mastoid cavity is inflamed.*

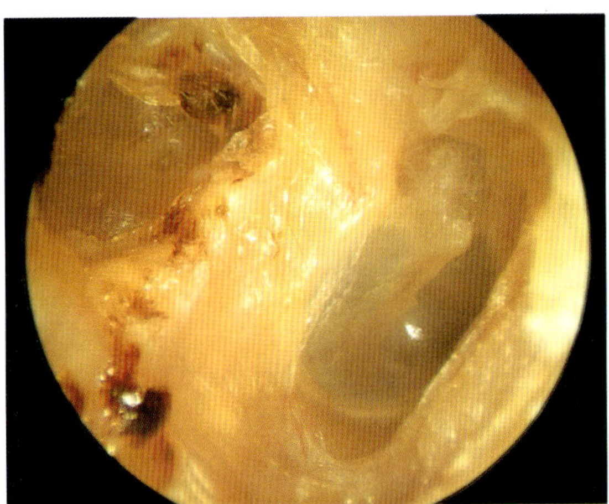

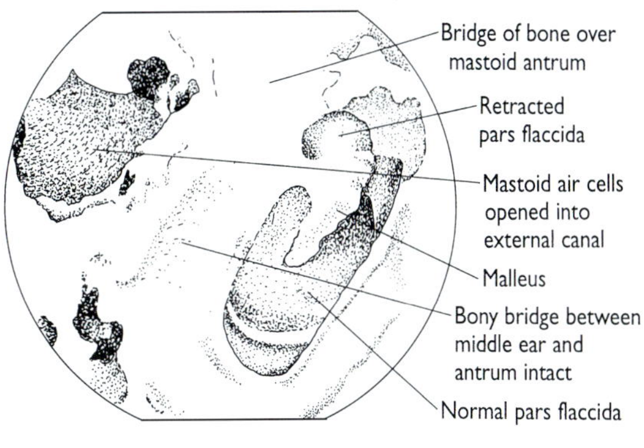

FIGURE 7.43 *Right inactive modified (Heath) mastoidectomy. The pars tensa is normal. The pars flaccida is retracted but inactive. Posteriorly the mastoid air cells have been surgically opened into the external canal by partial removal of the posterior canal wall. The bridge of bone over the incudal fossa and the mastoid antrum is normally removed in a modified radical mastoidectomy (and in an attico-antrostomy). It has not been removed in this case. There is no evidence of activity.*

always present with a discharge (Figure 7.50). When squamous epithelium is left behind an intact membrane or out of view in a closed mastoid air cell system, it forms a pearl, not unlike an inclusion cyst. This can progressively enlarge until it becomes clinically obvious or a complication such as ossicular disruption with a deterioration in hearing occurs. Variations can also occur that are uncommon in developed countries. Maggots can breed in a wet cavity in hot, humid environments (Figure 7.51). Tuberculosis and carcinoma (see below) have to be considered in all countries if the appearance is atypical or does not settle with conventional therapy. Biopsy is then indicated.

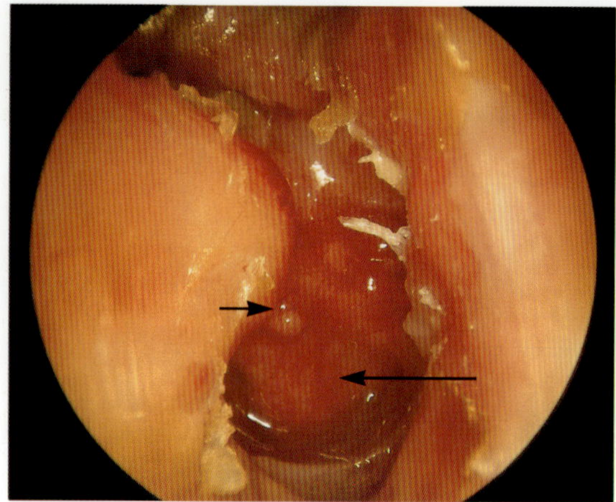

FIGURE 7.44 *Right active mucosal disease in modified radical mastoidectomy. There is no obvious residual pars tensa or flaccida. The middle ear mucosa (long arrow) is grossly inflamed. The stapes is the only residual ossicle (short arrow). The mastoid cavity is difficult to assess because of inadequate lowering of the posterior canal wall. The antrum only has been exposed and there is almost certainly activity in the mastoid air cells out of view.*

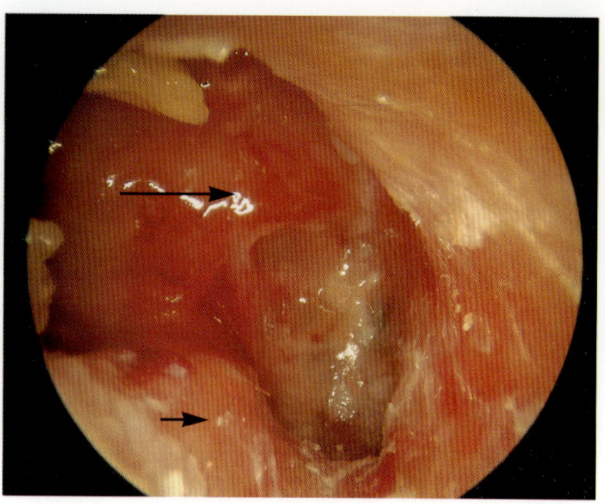

FIGURE 7.45 *Right active mucosal disease in modified radical mastoidectomy. In contrast to Figure 7.44, the activity is primarily in the mastoid cavity, the pars tensa probably being intact and the middle ear essentially inactive. The posterior canal wall has been lowered more than in Figure 7.44 (short arrow) but the cavity is lined by grossly hypertrophied mucosa (long arrow).*

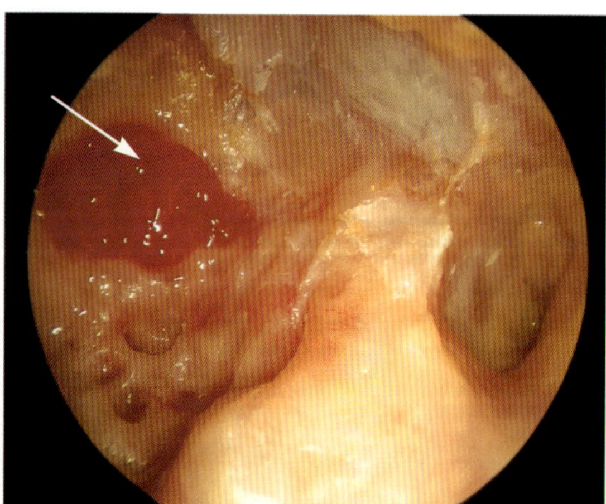

FIGURE 7.46 *Right active mucosal disease in modified radical mastoidectomy. The activity in this ear is from granulation tissue in the mastoid cavity (arrowed). The pars tensa is intact.*

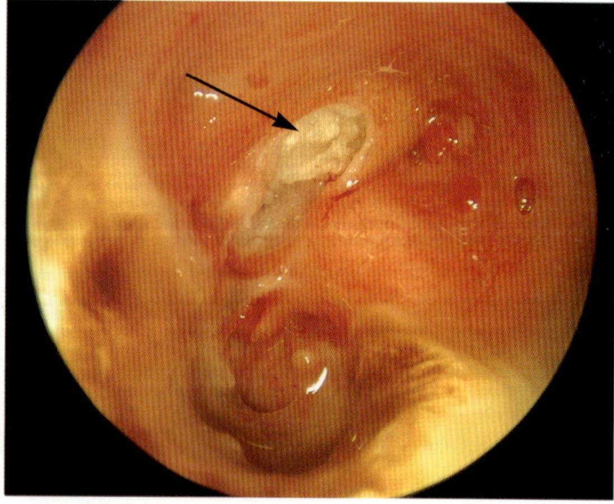

FIGURE 7.47 *Left active modified radical mastoidectomy with residual squamous disease (cholesteatoma). This ear is obviously active, there being mucosal disease in both the middle ear and mastoid cavity. In addition, superiorly in the cavity, there is squamous epithelial debris (arrowed) in a retraction pocket in an air cell.*

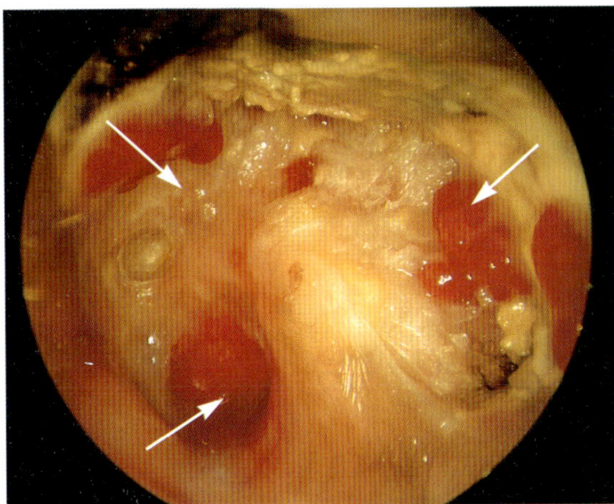

FIGURE 7.48 *Left active modified radical mastoidectomy with residual squamous disease (cholesteatoma). This ear is active with pus and squamous debris. Although there are granulations (arrows) in the middle ear, antrum and mastoid cavity, the epithelial debris arises from the squamous epithelial lining of the cavity and antrum.*

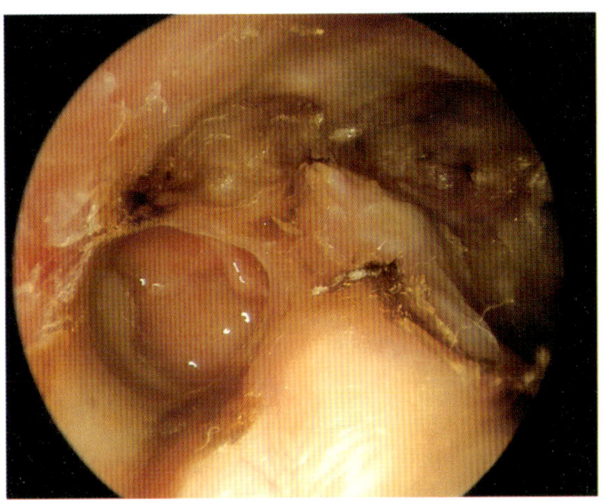

FIGURE 7.49 *Left active radical mastoidectomy. The pars tensa is absent and there is obvious active mucosal middle ear disease. The cavity appears dry but is lined by a crust and there is some retained debris. If this were to be removed there may or may not be active squamous disease.*

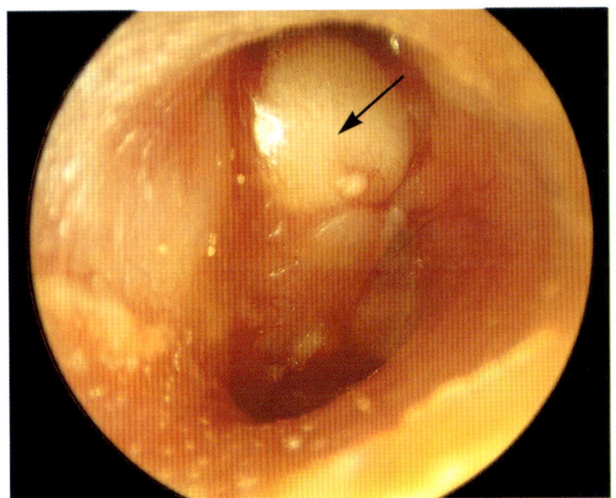

FIGURE 7.50 *Recurrent cholesteatoma in right atticotomy. There is a bony defect in the attic which is covered by a membrane, the result of a surgical graft of fascia. Behind this (arrowed) there is a white rounded mass which is a residual cholesteatomatous pearl.*

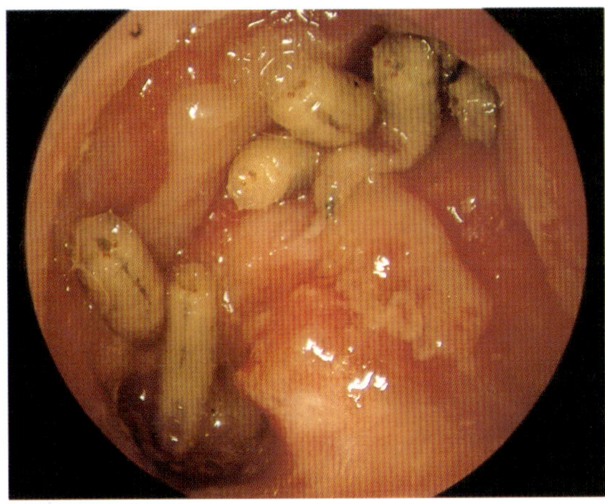

FIGURE 7.51 *Maggots in a left modified radical mastoidectomy.*

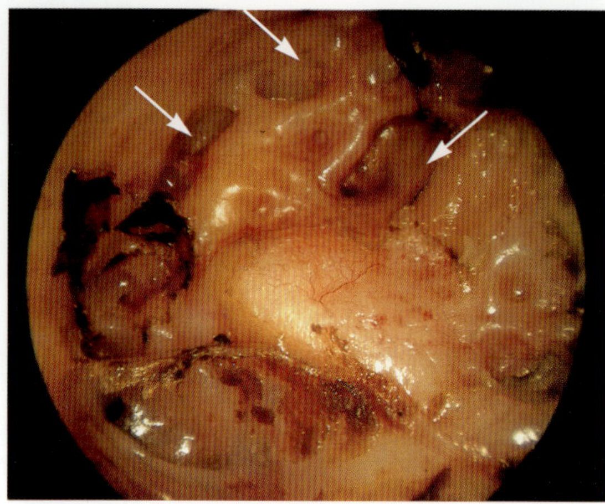

FIGURE 7.52 *Left inactive modified radical mastoidectomy. The lining of the mastoid cavity is inactive but retracted into multiple residual air cells (arrows). These could retain debris. The pars tensa is intact.*

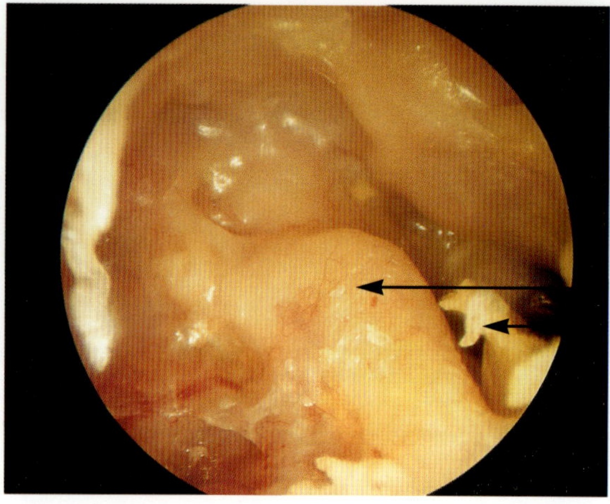

FIGURE 7.53 *Left active modified radical mastoidectomy. There is activity in the mastoid cavity sump (short arrow). This is due to the high residual posterior canal wall (long arrow) preventing migration of the epithelial lining out the canal.*

Management – general

After thorough aural toilet, it should be possible to assess which anatomical areas are active. All crusts need to be removed because frequently there is active disease behind them. Even though the indication for creating an open mastoid cavity is usually active squamous disease, residual activity is most frequently from mucosal disease either in the middle ear cleft (Figure 7.44), in the cavity itself (Figure 7.45), or very frequently both. Granulation tissue or small polyps are frequent, and provided they are not over the fallopian (facial) canal or in the oval or round windows then careful avulsion or cautery can be helpful (Figure 7.46).

Topical antibiotic and steroid drops or sprays can be used to settle active mucosal disease in a mastoid cavity, but this is, unfortunately, infrequently achieved. The long-term answer is revision surgery.

Management – revision surgery

Revision surgery for a modified radical mastoid cavity that remains active is tailored to each patient's specific problems. A decision as to which of the following procedures is most appropriate often has to await a fuller assessment under anaesthesia when the ear has been opened.

- Meatoplasty: Whenever an open mastoid cavity is created, the external auditory canal requires to be enlarged by removal of conchal cartilage. The amount of removal depends on the final size of the cavity. In cavities that continue to discharge or build up debris there is almost invariably an inadequate meatoplasty.

- Mastoid obliteration: In large cavities consideration should always be given to reducing their size by obliteration with bone pâté or muscle flaps. This can reduce the required size of the meatoplasty and also the necessity to lower any further a high posterior canal wall. Figure 7.52 shows a modified radical cavity with multiple 'nooks and crannies' that could retain debris though this is not the case at present. Further exenteration of these residual air cells would create a very large cavity which would be better being obliterated.

- Lowering posterior canal wall: The residual ridge over the facial nerve should be smooth, gradually building up to the floor of the canal and have no mastoid sump behind it. In many ears (Figures 7.42, 7.44, 7.46, 7.48 and especially 7.53) the posterior canal

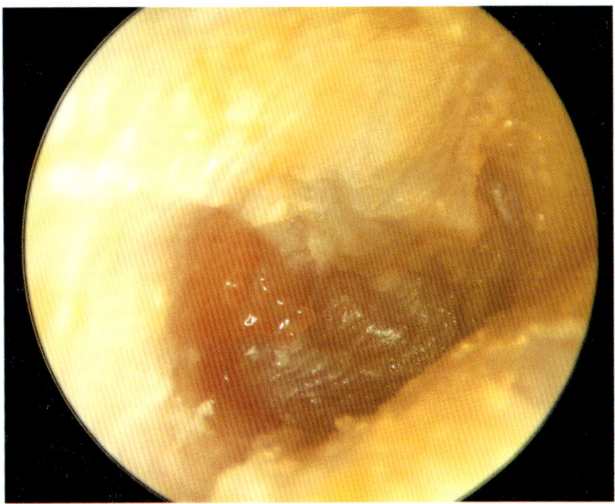

FIGURE 7.54 *Right granular myringitis. There is pus in the canal but the pars tensa appears intact. However, there is granulation tissue arising from it posteriorly extending on to the adjacent canal wall. The intactness of the pars tensa can be confirmed by pneumatic otoscopy or tympanometry.*

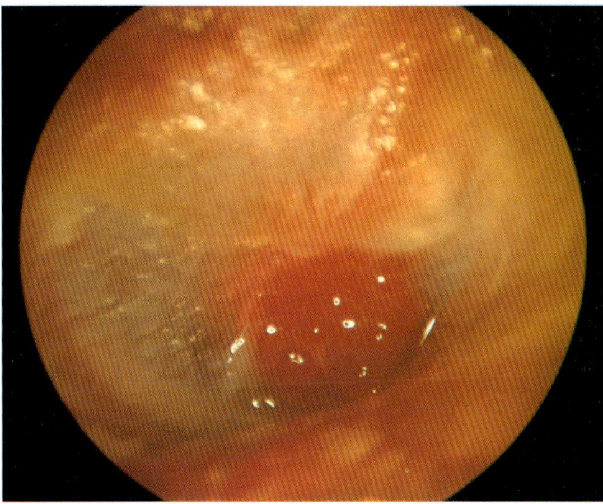

FIGURE 7.55 *Right granular myringitis. The ear is active, there being pus in the canal and granulation tissue inferiorly on an apparently intact pars tensa.*

wall has not been lowered sufficiently. This prevents the squamous epithelium from migrating satisfactorily out the canal. Debris is retained rather than shed. An alternative to totally lowering the posterior canal wall is to obliterate any sump.

- Mastoid lining: The aim is to have a squamous epithelial lined mastoid cavity which is naturally self-cleansing due to epithelial migration. After surgical removal of all diseased mucosa, the residual air cells can be covered with a free graft or a pedicled flap of fascia. This encourages fibro-osseous sclerosis of the residual mastoid air cells and gives a good bed for the squamous epithelium to migrate over.
- Closure of middle ear cleft: Active middle ear mucosal disease is best dealt with by grafting of the pars tensa to create an enclosed middle ear air-containing space.

SPECIALIST – RECONSIDER DIAGNOSIS

Though active chronic otitis media is the most frequent cause of an ear discharge apart from otitis externa, there are other diagnoses to consider.

GRANULAR MYRINGITIS

Granular myringitis should be suspected if the discharge comes from granulation tissue on an apparently intact pars tensa (Figures 7.54 and 7.55). In some cases there is a small perforation with granulation tissue on the surrounding squamous epithelium. The intactness or otherwise of the tympanic membrane can usually be assessed by pneumatic otoscopy.

The aetiology of granular myringitis is uncertain. There is debate as to whether it starts as an area of granulation tissue on the squamous epithelium of the pars tensa that sometimes results in a small perforation. The alternative is that it starts as active middle ear disease which results in a small perforation with resultant granulation tissue around it. Treatment is with topical medication, most usually some form of cautery after thorough aural toilet. Topical steroid and antibiotic eardrops are an alternative therapy.

CARCINOMA OF THE MIDDLE EAR

Fortunately carcinoma of the middle ear is relatively uncommon but should be suspected if an ear with a long-standing history of discharge

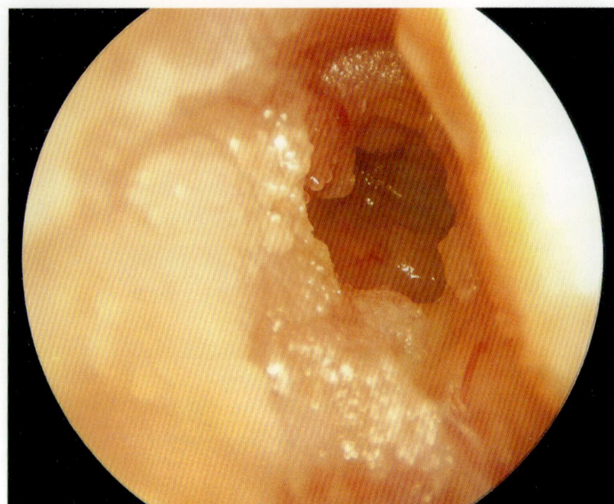

FIGURE 7.56 *Carcinoma of right ear. The granulation tissue on the canal wall and middle ear is unlike that most frequently seen in active chronic otitis media. Under these circumstances biopsy is essential. No anatomical landmarks are identifiable.*

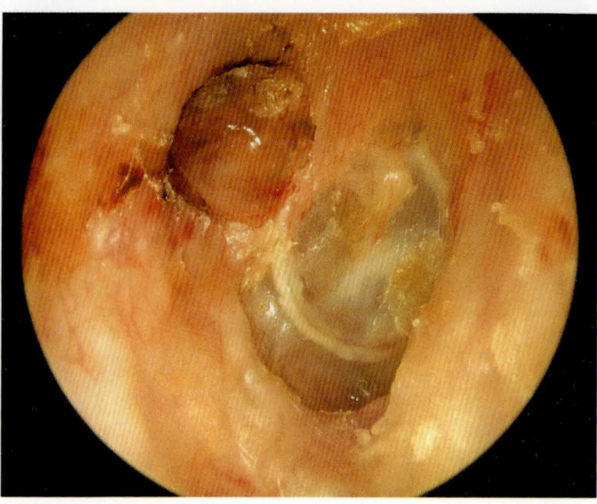

FIGURE 7.57 *Radionecrosis of right ear. In this ear there is a bony defect of the posterior canal wall, a bone sequestrum having been extruded.*

from COM becomes uncomfortable. Otoscopically there is exuberant granulation tissue out of keeping with that expected in active COM (Figure 7.56).

Management

After confirmatory biopsy and CT scanning to assess the carcinoma's extent, ablative surgery with radiotherapy occasionally is curative.

RADIONECROSIS

Radionecrosis of the temporal bone is rare, but can occur many years after radiotherapy given to structures near the ear such as the parotid. Its presentation is similar to active COM (Figure 7.57) and may not be thought of unless a past history is elucidated. The necrotic bone may sometimes be apparent.

BENIGN NECROTISING OTITIS EXTERNA

The cause of this rare condition is unknown. Pathologically there is a bone sequestra which ulcerates through the skin (Figure 7.58) usually on the floor of the canal.

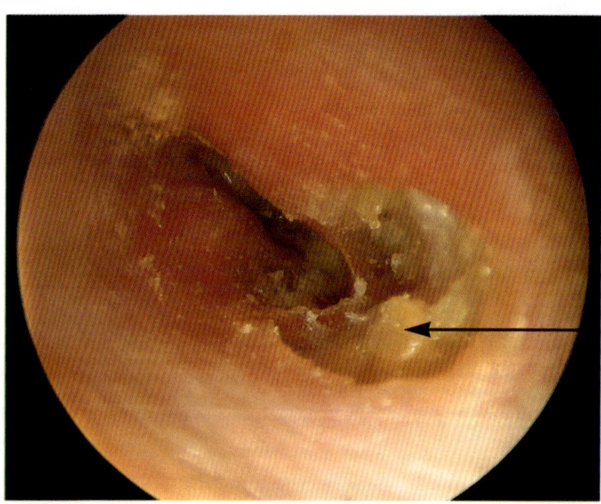

FIGURE 7.58 *Benign necrotising otitis externa (left). A bone sequestrum (arrow) is present in the gross defect in the postero-inferior canal wall.*

CHAPTER 8

EAR TRAUMA

The ear can be traumatised in many ways but in general each mechanism of injury tends to affect specific areas. The mechanism of injury is usually apparent from the history and the damage sustained is usually evident on otoscopy.

SELF TRAUMA – EXTERNAL CANAL INJURY

Perhaps the most common ear injury is self-inflicted with a match, cotton bud, ballpoint pen clip or hairpin. Most frequently the canal skin is broken (Figure 8.1) but tears of the tympanic membrane can also occur. Unfortunately the tip of an ear syringe can also be traumatic (Figure 8.2). Fortunately, natural repair is normal.

PRESSURE TRAUMA – EXTERNAL AND MIDDLE EAR INJURY

An *acute* change of pressure difference between tympanic membrane and middle ear such as occurs in flying or going deep underwater will mainly cause otalgia. If the pressure difference is sustained, the tympanic membrane may become injected and have

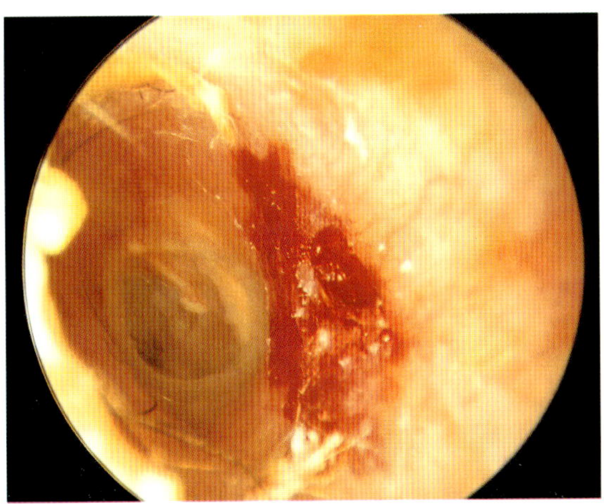

FIGURE 8.1 *Trauma to (left) external auditory canal due to patient poking.*

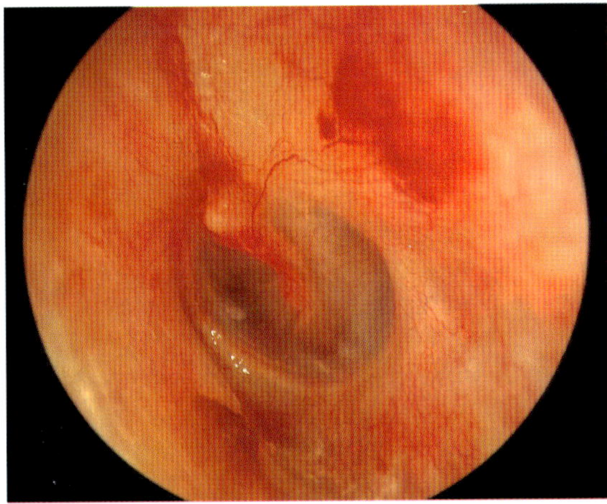

FIGURE 8.2 *Trauma to (left) external auditory canal due to tip of ear syringe. There is an area of haemorrhage in the posterosuperior canal skin. In addition there is a tympanic 'flush' of the canal and tympanic membrane. This is a normal reaction following syringing.*

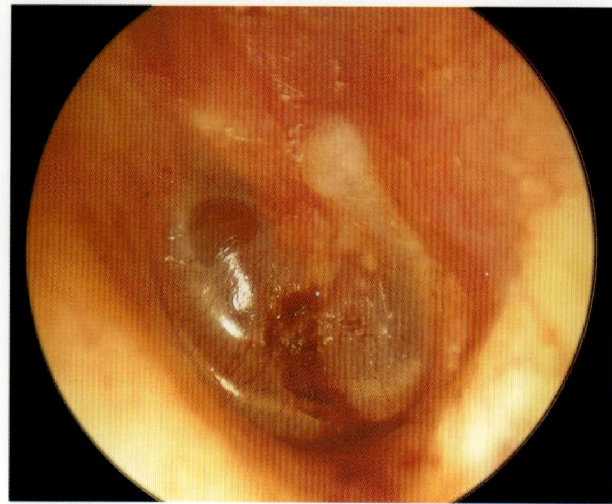

FIGURE 8.3 *Diving barotrauma (left). The canal skin and tympanic membrane are hyperaemic but the main finding is that the tympanic membrane is retracted and there is red haemorrhagic fluid in the middle ear.*

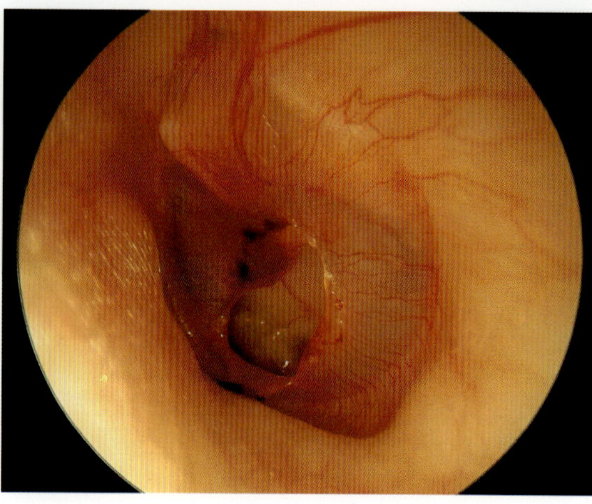

FIGURE 8.4 *Tympanic membrane perforation (left) secondary to blow on ear. At the inferior edge of the perforation, part of the torn tympanic membrane is everted.*

areas of haemorrhage within it (Figure 8.3). Rarely the tympanic membrane may rupture but this is more common following a slap to the ear or an explosion (Figure 8.4). Almost invariably natural healing of such injuries occurs.

TEMPORAL BONE FRACTURE – EXTERNAL, MIDDLE AND INNER EAR INJURY

If the side of the head is injured with sufficient force, a temporal bone fracture can result. Usually there is blood in the external auditory canal and the fracture line may be seen on the roof of the external auditory canal (Figure 8.5). If there is bony displacement, a step may be visible.

The presence of blood in the external auditory canal following a head injury is diagnostic of a temporal bone fracture provided it has not come from outside the ear. It is generally held that the canal should not be cleaned if there is a fracture because of the risk of introducing infection. If the tympanic membrane is seen, it may be intact or torn in line with the fracture. If intact, the middle ear will be full of blood and CSF which has a fairly classic appear-

ance (Figure 8.6). If the tympanic membrane is torn, there may be an obvious CSF leak, as well as there being blood in the canal. Whatever the findings, if a fracture is suspected prophylactic antibiotics are given to lessen the chance of intracranial infection. Most CSF leaks cease spontaneously, but if they last longer than ten days, it is usual to surgically repair the dural defect.

Once the patient has recovered sufficiently the hearing should be assessed audiometrically. A conductive impairment may be due to the middle ear fluid, ossicular disruption or both. Follow up will distinguish between these as the impairment associated with ossicular disruption will not resolve. A sensorineural impairment can also occur due to cochlear damage but rarely recovers. Facial movement should be assessed as soon as practical, as the facial nerve may be damaged by the fracture and require repair.

SURGERY – MIDDLE AND INNER EAR INJURY

Any form of ear surgery is by definition traumatic but usually healing occurs without

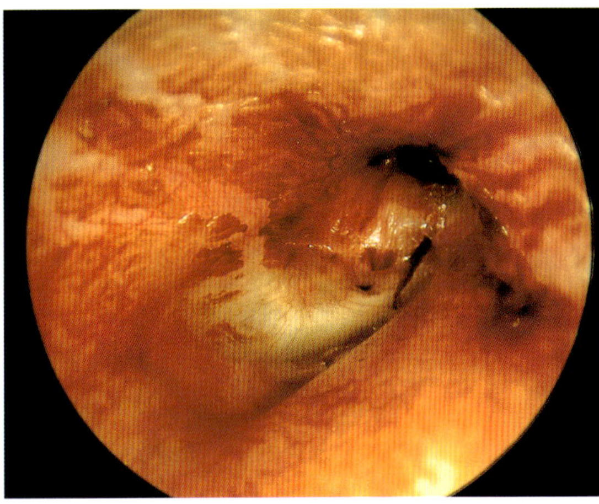

FIGURE 8.5 *Temporal bone fracture (right). Haemorrhage is from a fracture which runs along roof of the external auditory canal.*

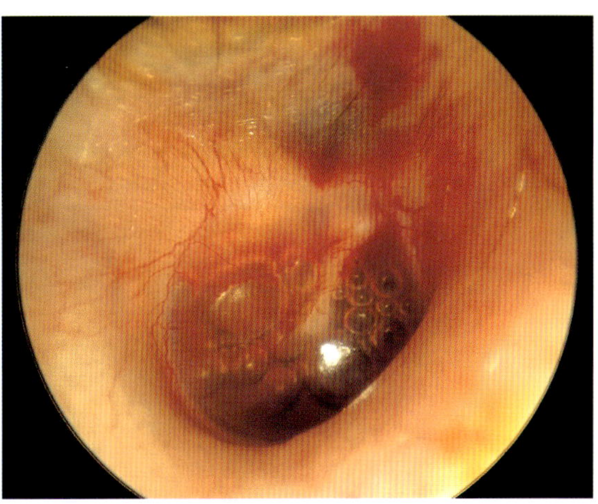

FIGURE 8.6 *Temporal bone fracture with blood stained CSF and air (bubbles) in right middle ear. Fracture line as Figure 8.5 on roof of external canal.*

problems. Granulation tissue can occur along incision lines, particularly if a gap has been left. This is particularly likely in open mastoid surgery. Inclusion cysts of squamous epithelium (Figure 8.7) mainly occur in incision lines or where flaps have been raised and squamous epithelium inadvertently buried. Surgical removal is not difficult.

Unfortunately, more severe damage sometimes occurs. A conductive impairment may arise if an intact ossicular chain is disrupted to remove disease. An ossiculoplasty can help mitigate this. A sensorineural impairment and/or vertigo may occur if the stapes is moved excessively or the inner ear opened at the oval window or a semicircular canal. A facial palsy may result from trauma to an exposed nerve which may have occurred naturally, been produced by disease or secondary to surgery. CSF leaks can occur due to dural tears, followed sometimes by secondary intracranial infection.

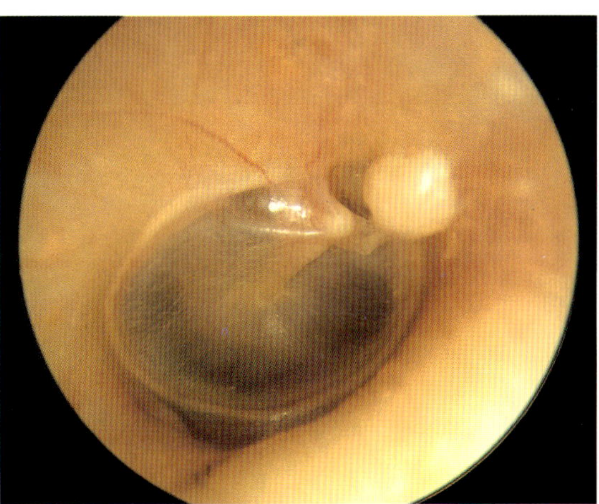

FIGURE 8.7 *Inclusion cyst in right attic.*

CHAPTER 9

TECHNIQUES OF EXAMINATION
(INCLUDING OTOSCOPY, AURAL TOILET AND HEARING ASSESSMENT)

All patients with otological symptoms require otoscopy and their hearing assessed. It is usual to start with otoscopy because in some instances wax and debris need to be removed. This in itself may improve the hearing.

OTOSCOPY

INSTRUMENTS

An otoscope (auriscope) is the basic instrument required. Otoscopes can vary in:

(a) Power   disposable or rechargeable batteries
           mains transformer
(b) Light   tungsten
           halogen (three times brighter)
(c) Head   closed to allow pneumatic otoscopy
           open to allow instrumentation
(d) Speculum   detachable
           sleeved over nose cone

The decision as to which otoscope to use is usually made for one, there being only one type available. The strength of the battery should always be checked, the most common reason for a poor view being insufficient light.

TECHNIQUE

Having examined the pinna for abnormalities and operation scars (Figures 9.1 and 9.2), the

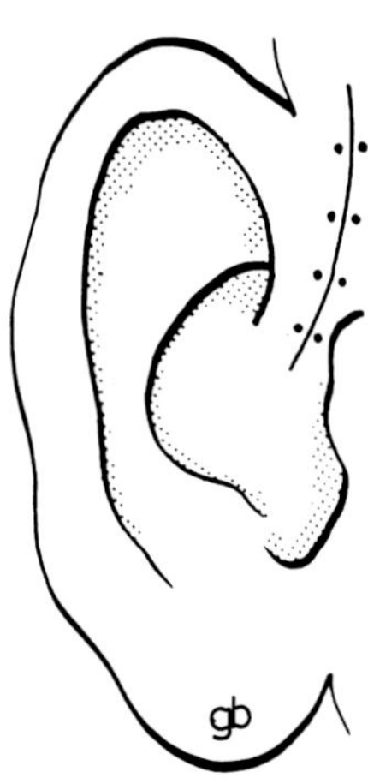

FIGURE 9.1 *Endaural incision. Right ear.*

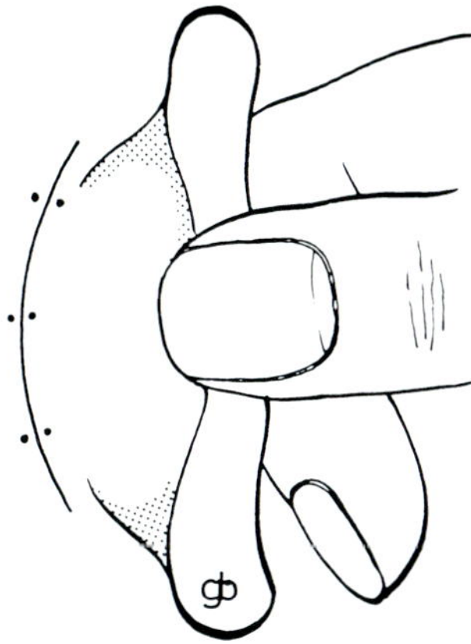

FIGURE 9.2 *Postauricular incision. Right ear.*

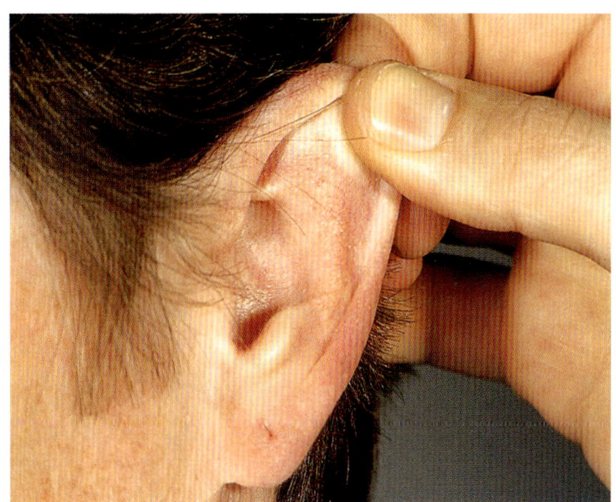

FIGURE 9.3 *Positioning of ear for otoscopy.*

largest speculum that the canal can take is selected and fitted to the otoscope. As the patient's head has to be held still, and because the normal external auditory canal is angled, the pinna is pulled posterosuperiorly with one hand which straightens the canal (Figure 9.3). The otoscope is best held with the fingers like a pen rather than in the palm of the hand. The speculum is inserted to allow a view of the canal and tympanic membrane. This requires looking in different directions.

If a patient has had a previous operation, the type of scar (if any) increases the likelihood of certain abnormalities being detected (Table 9.1). If an abnormality is identified with an otoscope, in most cases greater magnification will give additional information. Formerly magnification was achieved with a Seigle's speculum but today the operating microscope is more frequently used. The patient can be seated or lying on a couch, the latter being preferred if instrumentation is necessary. Oval ended metal specula are frequently used, their advantage being that they more naturally fit the shape of the canal than the round ones on an otoscope. Alternatively split specula may be used.

Technique of pneumatic otoscopy

The object here is to hermetically close the external auditory canal and assess whether the tympanic membrane is mobile when the canal pressure is altered. There are two main ways to do this. The simplest is with a closed otoscope

Table 9.1 *Relationship between site of operation scar and likely operation and diagnosis*

Scars	Likely preop. condition	Potential operation	Potential abnormality
None	OME	Myringotomy and grommet	HOM
			Retraction
			COM
Postauricular	COM	Myringoplasty/tympanoplasty	HOM
		Cortical (simple) mastoidectomy	HOM or COM
		Modified radical mastoidectomy	Open cavity
Endaural	COM	Myringotomy/tympanoplasty	HOM
		Attico-antrostomy	Open cavity
	Otosclerosis	Stapedotomy/stapedectomy	HOM

OME, otitis media with effusion; COM, chronic otitis media; HOM, healed otitis media.

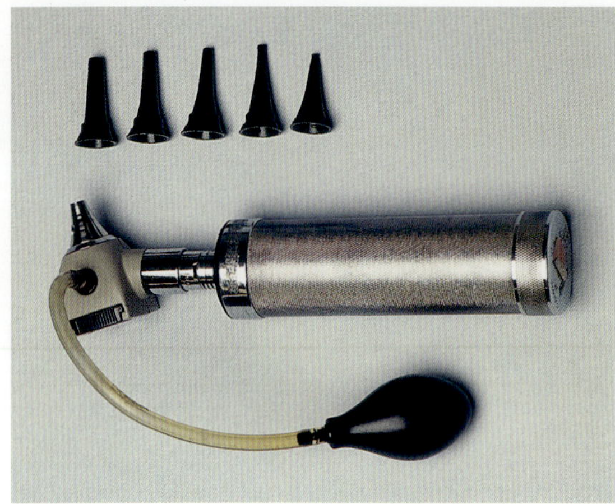

FIGURE 9.4 *Closed pneumatic otoscope.*

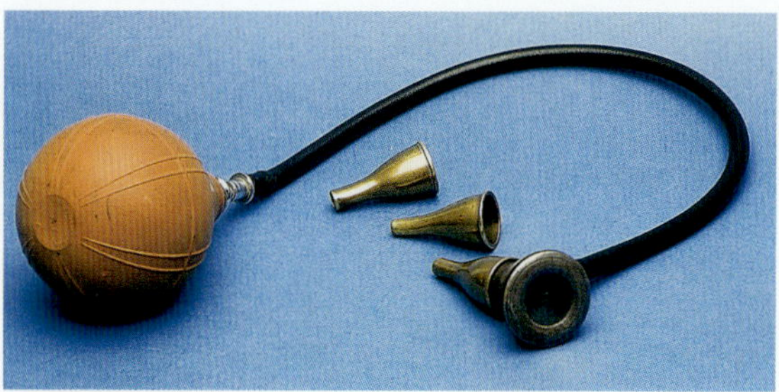

FIGURE 9.5 *Seigle's pneumatic otoscope.*

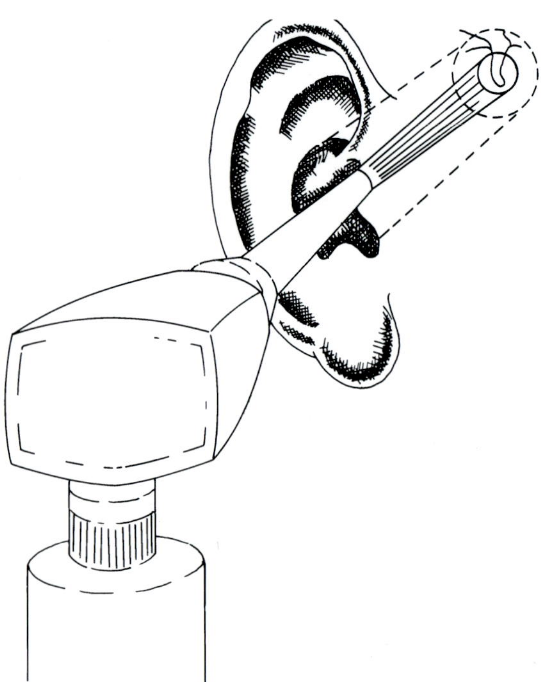

FIGURE 9.6 *Illustration of limited view obtained via a speculum.*

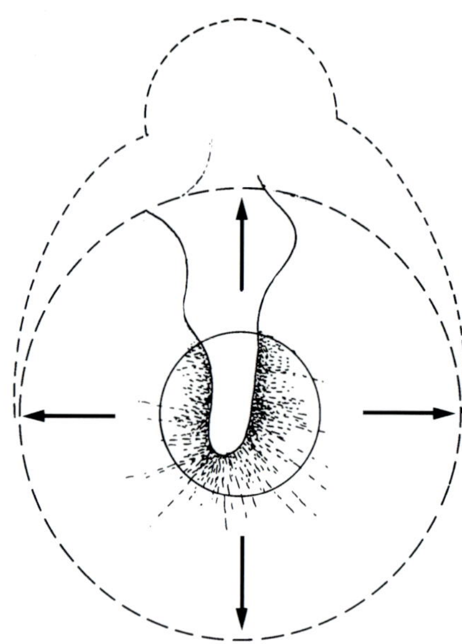

FIGURE 9.7 *Illustration of how, by moving the line of view, an area larger than the central circle can be viewed in a speculum.*

(Figure 9.4). This, when snugly inserted in the canal, creates an enclosed air system whose pressure can be altered by pressed the attached rubber bulb. If the tympanic membrane is seen to move, this virtually excludes middle ear fluid.

Unfortunately, an apparently immobile tympanic membrane may be due to an air seal not being obtained in the canal as well as middle ear fluid. A better seal is likely to be obtained with an oval speculum as part of a closed Seigle's system (Figure 9.5). If this is used with a headlight, the glass cover is a magnifying lens, but when used with a microscope, plain glass is all that is required.

Limitations of the hand-held otoscope and microscope

The hand-held otoscope produces a parallel beam of light which illuminates the area onto

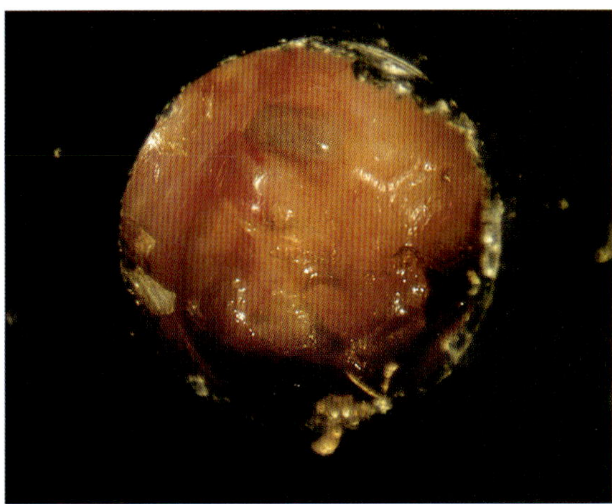

FIGURE 9.8 *Limited view of attic obtained via a speculum.*

the anterior bulge of the temporomandibular joint. Mastoid cavities with a narrow meatus or high residual posterior canal wall may also be missed.

The entire area of the tympanic membrane needs to be systematically assessed otherwise failure to observe an area may lead to misdiagnosis. For example, if the attic is not visualised a cholesteatoma or a mastoid cavity may be missed (Figures 9.8 and 9.9). Similar principles apply to otomicroscopy as this is also performed through an aural speculum. With both these methods the otoscopist is required to piece together separate pictures to form an overall picture on which the diagnosis is made. When the area to be examined is large, as in a mastoid cavity, this makes conventional otoscopy more difficult.

In contrast, the Hopkins rod otoscope which was used for the photographs in this text has a wide-angled lens which usually allows the entire tympanic membrane and ear canal to be visualised (Figure 9.10). Bulges in the external canal such as the temporomandibular joint which may obscure the antero-inferior aspect of the tympanic membrane can be bypassed by introducing the rod further and allowing the wide-angled lens to view past the obstruction. These photographs make otoscopy seem easier than it is.

which it is directed. The narrower the speculum, the smaller the area of the canal or tympanic membrane that can be seen (Figure 9.6). The area examined can be increased by moving the angle of view around (Figure 9.7) but, unfortunately, the external canal is sensitive and patients will only tolerate a certain amount of movement. This may make certain areas difficult to view especially the area behind

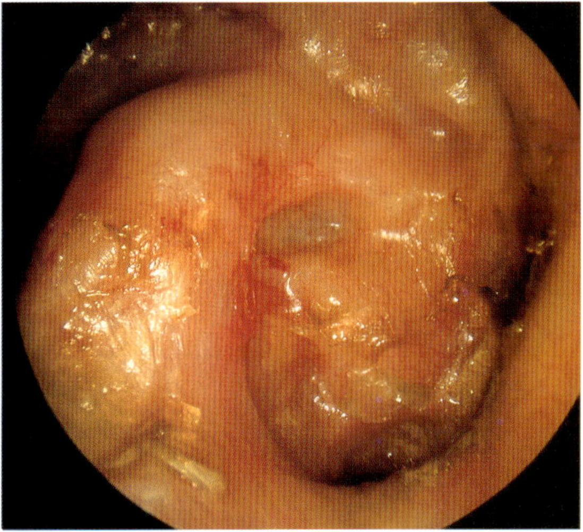

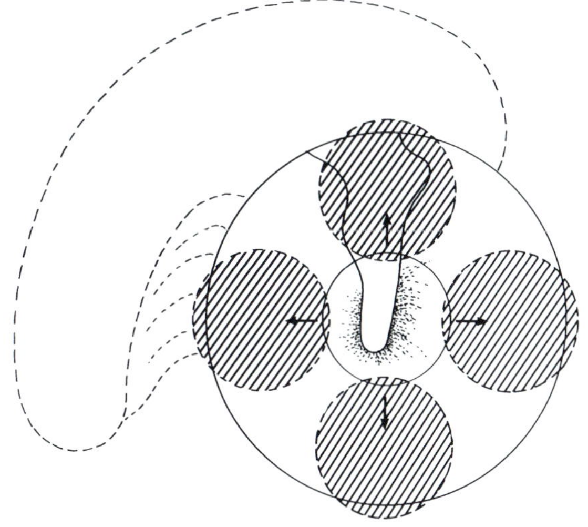

FIGURE 9.9a and b *Wider view of attic than in Figure 9.8 obtained by moving speculum. (a) Photograph taken with a rod scope. (b) Diagram of how such a picture is obtained by multiple views via a speculum.*

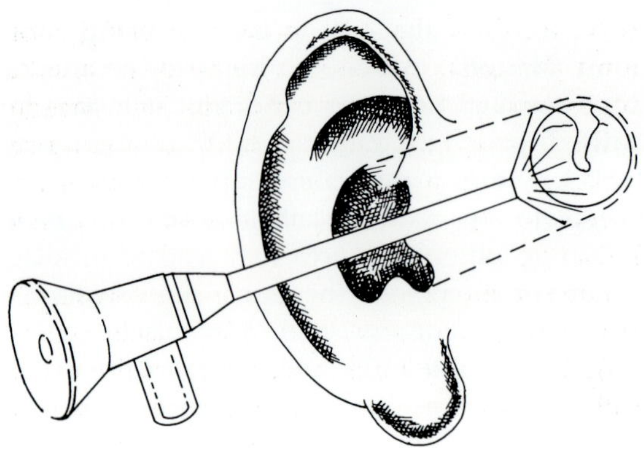

FIGURE 9.10 *Wide field of view obtained with a rod otoscope.*

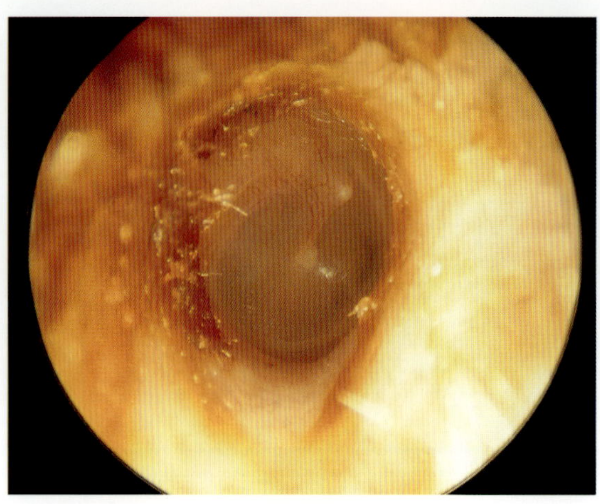

FIGURE 9.11 *Wax coating right canal. No need to remove.*

AURAL TOILET

A small amount of non-obstructive wax is normal (Figure 9.11) and only needs to be removed if the tympanic membrane cannot be fully visualised (Figure 9.12). The safest and easiest method for the non-specialist to remove wax is by syringing. If this is performed gently without causing discomfort, damage is unlikely even when a perforation pre-exists. Syringing is equally effective in clearing pus from the canal. Foreign bodies are also best removed by syringing.

Partially occlusive wax (Figures 9.12 and 9.13) is usually easy to syringe out. On the other hand, wax that has become impacted (Figure 9.14), often due to the use of cotton buds or an earmould of a hearing aid, may initially resist syringing. If this is thought likely, the wax should first be softened over two to three days with sodium bicarbonate ear drops before repeating syringing.

Syringing, if carried out correctly, is a safe procedure. If roughly inserted, the tip of the

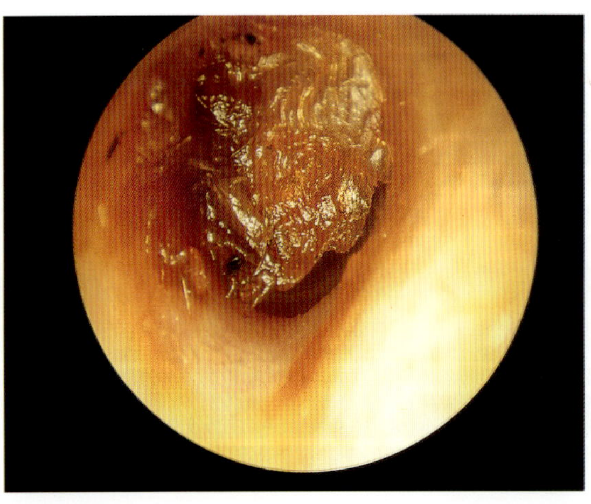

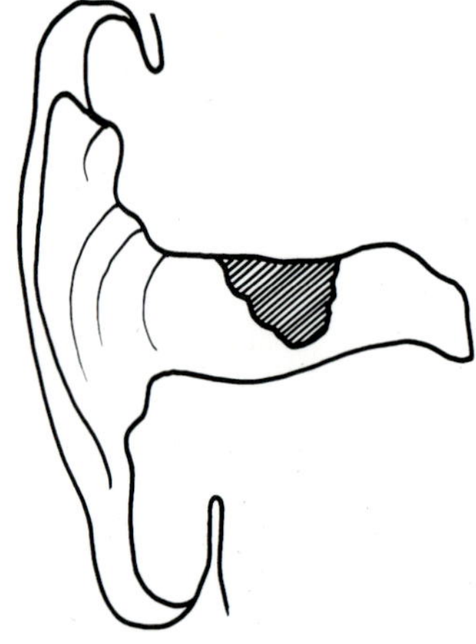

FIGURE 9.12a and b *Wax totally obscuring view of right tympanic membrane. Associated hearing impairment is unlikely.*

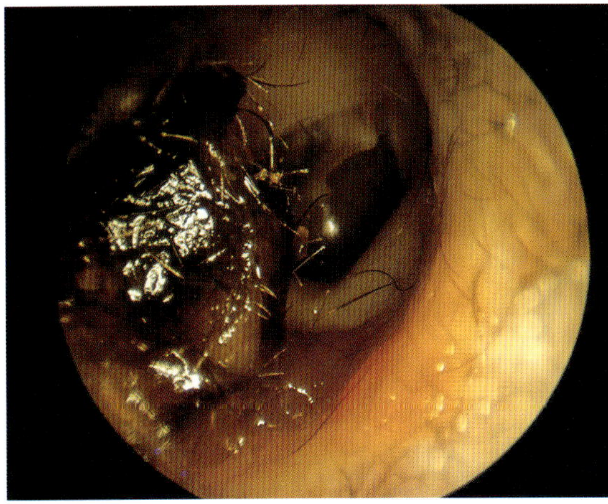

FIGURE 9.13 *Wax partially obscuring view of right tympanic membrane. This would not cause a hearing impairment.*

syringe may traumatise the canal skin (see Figure 8.2 page 75). Temporary dizziness may occur if the water is not at body temperature due to a caloric response. This can also occur if there is an open mastoid cavity even when the water temperature is correct.

TECHNIQUE

Ear syringes are made of plastic or metal. To this is attached a plastic or metal tip, which has to be firmly attached to prevent it being shot down the canal. An alternative is to use a soft, intravenous catheter or rubber tip. The syringe is filled with tap water at body temperature (checked with a thermometer) and excess air expelled. The plunger should move smoothly and not stick.

The pinna is pulled in a posterosuperior direction to straighten the canal (see Figure 9.3). The syringe tip is placed against the canal wall near the entrance and the water expelled (Figure 9.15). The stream should be aimed at and hit the canal wall rather than the tympanic membrane. The water will then go between it and the wax before hitting the tympanic membrane and flushing the wax out. If the wax proves resistant, otoscopy should identify the direction in which the syringe should point to bypass the wax and build up pressure behind it. Following syringing the canal should be dried with a cotton bud. Commercially made cotton ear buds are unsuitable as they tend to be too thick and the cotton wool woven so tightly that it can be traumatic. To make a cotton wool bud, a small piece of non-synthetic cotton wool is teased into a thin film and an orange stick placed halfway along it (Figure 9.16). The orange stick is rolled between the fingers to attach the cotton wool to the stick. The object

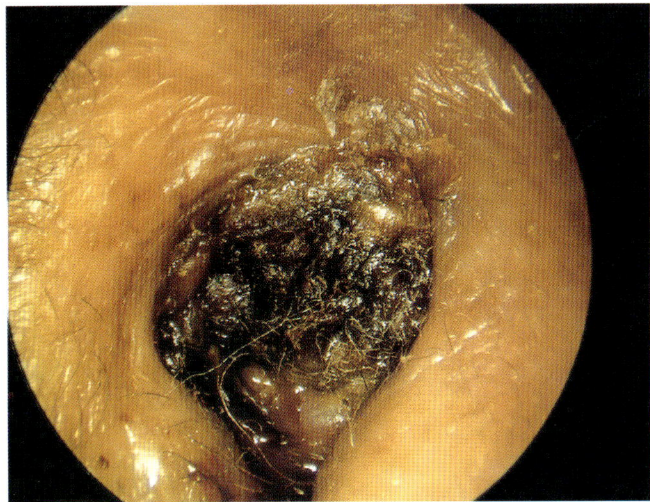

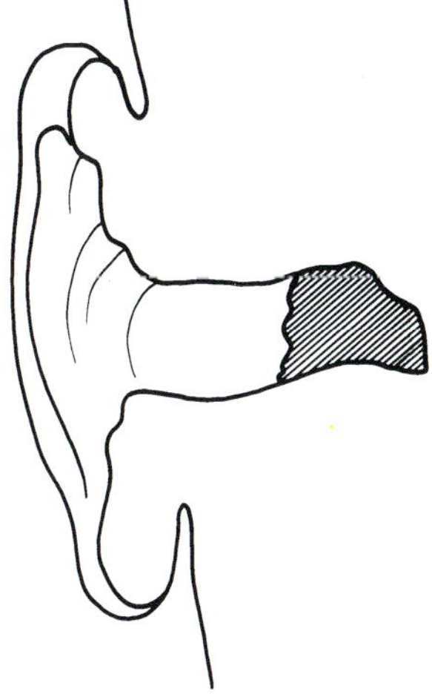

FIGURE 9.14a and b *Impacted wax against right tympanic membrane. Associated hearing impairment is likely.*

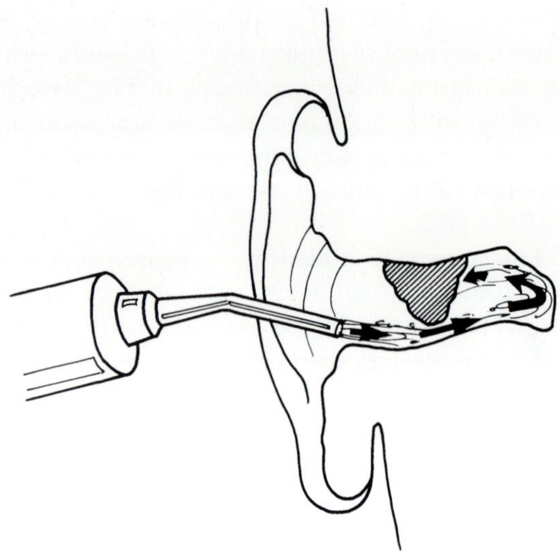

FIGURE 9.15 *Wax syringing. The water bypasses the wax and is reflected by the tympanic membrane to expel the wax.*

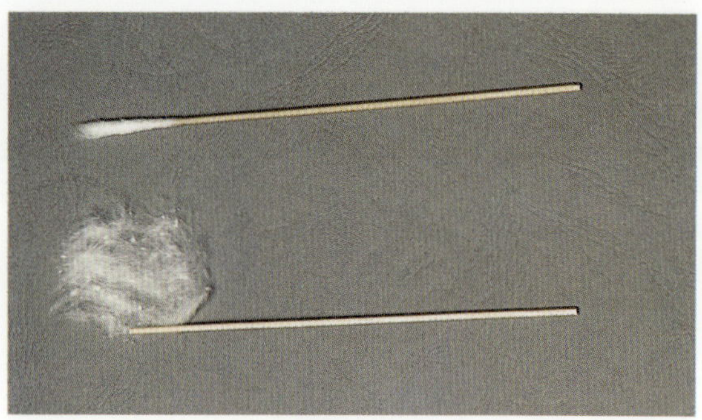

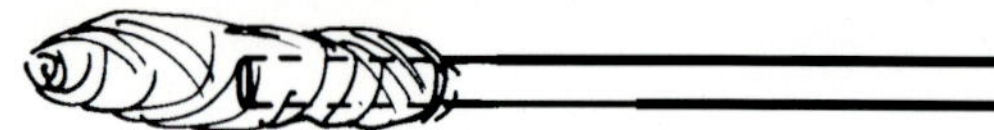

of placing the stick halfway up the bud is to allow the top half of the bud to be soft and atraumatic (Figure 9.17).

To mop the canal, this must first be straightened. The bud is held lightly between the forefinger and thumb and gently inserted into the canal (Figure 9.18). Following syringing this should remove any excess water. Otoscopy should then be repeated. It is normal for the canal skin and tympanic membrane to be slightly hyperaemic following syringing – a 'tympanic flush' (see Figure 8.2 page 75).

Where mopping is being performed to remove an aural discharge, this should be repeated until the cotton buds are dry and otoscopically there is no residual pus. Should there be any difficulties in syringing, the patient should be referred to a specialist.

Aural toilet – specialist

INSTRUMENTS

The specialist has the advantage of being able to perform aural toilet under direct vision. This can be with a headlight or a microscope. Every

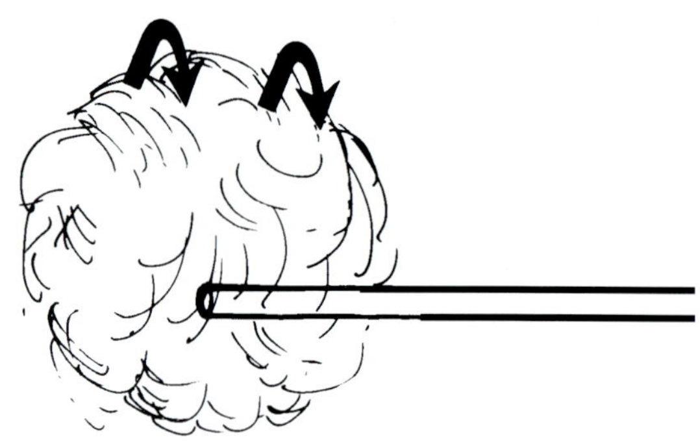

FIGURE 9.16a and b *Method of making a cotton bud.*

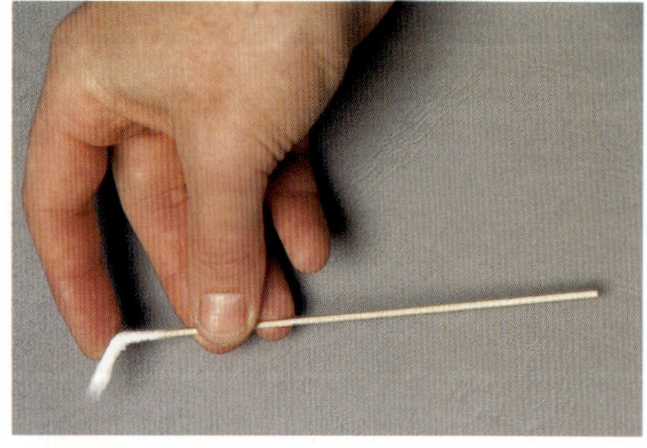

FIGURE 9.17 *Self-made cotton bud with atraumatic tip.*

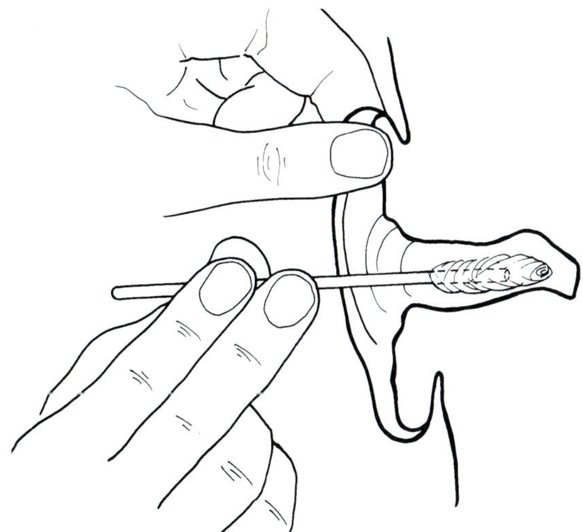

FIGURE 9.18 *Canal mopping with cotton bud.*

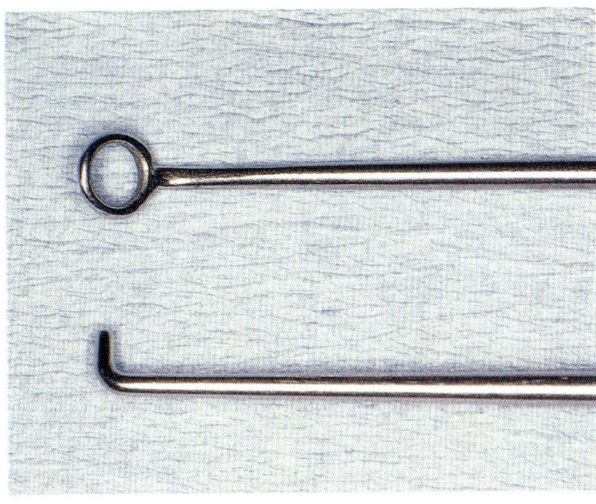

FIGURE 9.19 *Jobson–Horn probe (top). Wax hook (bottom).*

specialist has their favourite instruments. A Jobson–Horn probe (Figure 9.19) has a rounded end which is used to remove wax. The other end can be used with cotton wool as a cotton bud. The Jobson–Horn probe is not suitable for removing wax in the deep canal as slight head movement may cause injury. A wax hook with an angled, blunt end (Figure 9.19) can sometimes be used to remove impacted wax as a complete plug.

Wax that is difficult to remove should be initially softened and syringed out as much as possible. Thereafter, in most instances microscopic suction removes the remainder. However, several sessions may be required to totally remove impacted wax or debris in some patients.

Technique of microsuction

As the noise of the suction can be frightening, what is about to happen should be explained to the patient. Preferably they will be lying on an examination table and the otoscopist should be comfortably seated (Figure 9.20). The largest speculum that fits snugly is selected and a large sucker is used to clean out the outer canal, care being taken to avoid touching the canal wall as

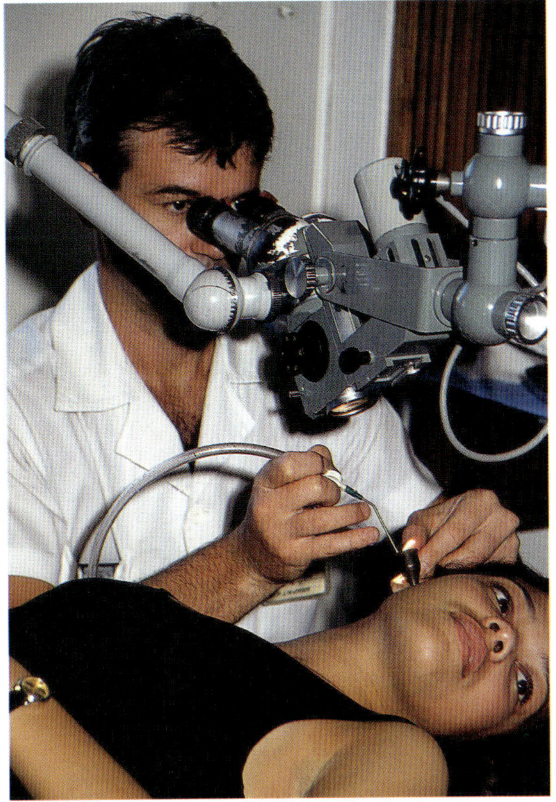

FIGURE 9.20 *Correct position of otoscopist.*

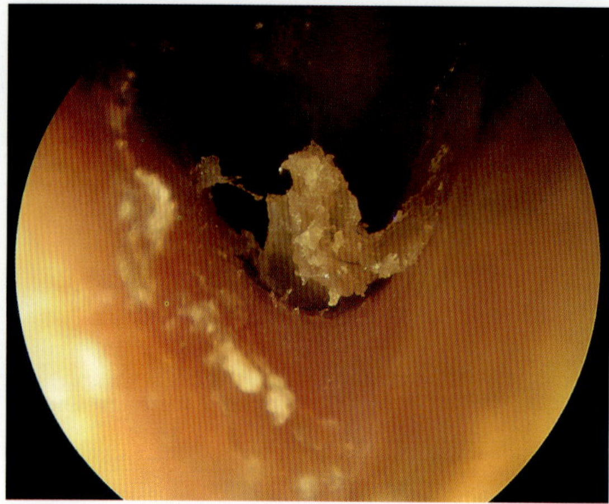

FIGURE 9.21 *Hardened keratinous debris, most easily removed with microforceps.*

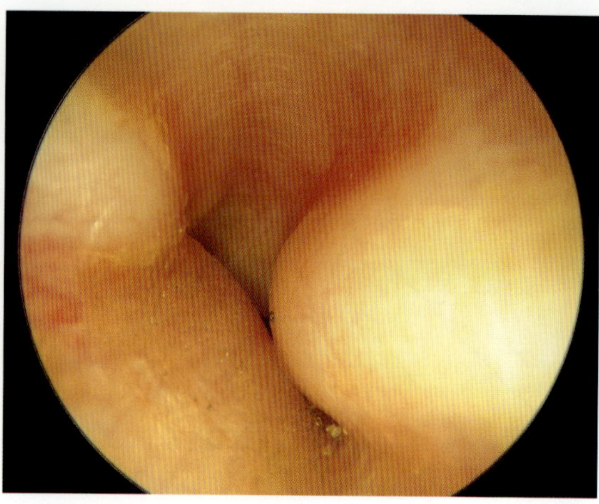

FIGURE 9.22 *Multiple exostosis of right external auditory canal. One exostosis is anterior and two are posterior.*

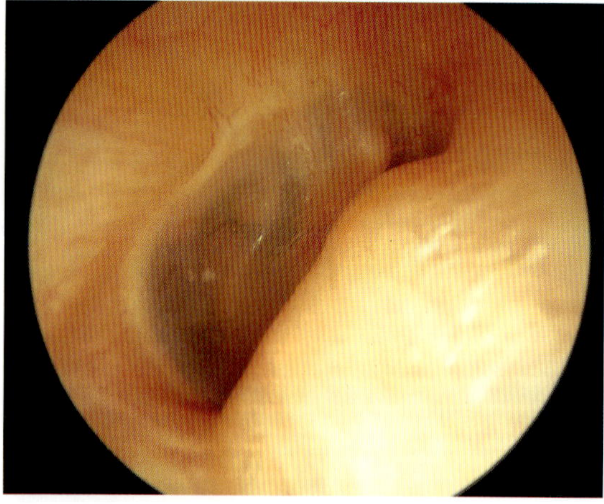

FIGURE 9.23 *Single anterior exostosis of right external auditory canal.*

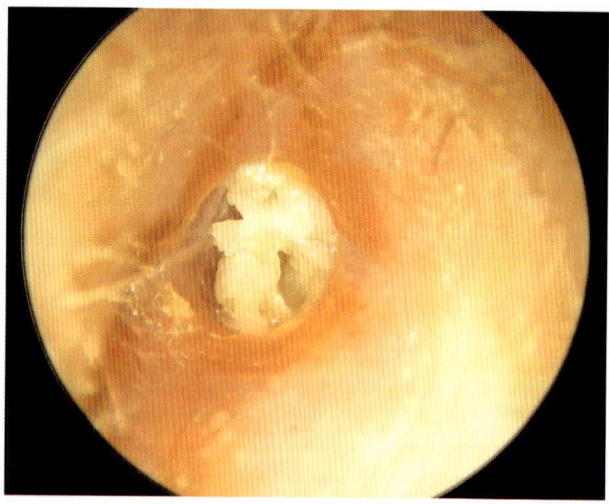

FIGURE 9.24 *Impacted squames in the deep bony canal, behind a partial stenosis. Right ear.*

this may be extremely tender. Deeper down the canal, greater care is required and finer suckers are selected. Suction of the tympanic membrane can usually be performed without discomfort, but touching the middle ear mucosa can be sensitive. Particular care should be taken to avoid touching the ossicular chain.

On occasions hardened discharge or debris (Figure 9.21) can be more easily removed with microforceps. Crusts or discharge in the attic must always be removed as they may conceal an underlying cholesteatoma (see Figures 7.28, 7.29 and 7.30, page 63).

SPECIALIST PROBLEMS

EXOSTOSES

Exostoses form in the deep bony canal in response to prolonged exposure to cold. Thus

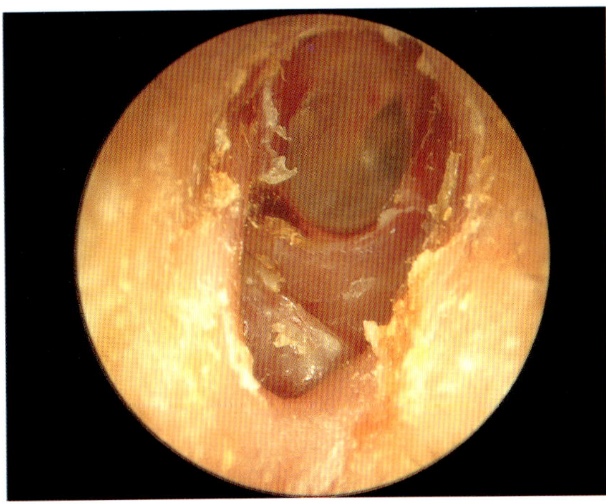

FIGURE 9.25 *External canal keratoma has been removed but expansion of the deep right bony canal remains.*

they are common in cold water sports enthusiasts like swimmers, sailors or surfers. Usually there is one growth anteriorly and two posteriorly (Figure 9.22) but on occasions they can be single (Figure 9.23). The majority of exostoses are asymptomatic being a chance finding on otoscopy and require no management. Some impede the normal migration of squamous epithelium out of the canal and then present with a hearing impairment due to a blocked canal. Others predispose to otitis externa. Surgical removal is relatively simple.

KERATOSIS OBTURANS

Keratosis obturans is relatively rare but can present in two different ways.

Deep canal obstruction by keratin

Desquamated epithelium, and occasionally wax, collects and impacts in the deep bony external canal behind a partial stenosis (Figure 9.24). A secondary otitis externa develops which causes the external canal skin to become oedematous compounding the obstruction.

External auditory canal keratoma

In these cases there appears to be an abnormal migration of epithelium out of the deep meatus. The desquamated epithelium forms

into a ball which is ever expanding and eventually causes erosion of the deep bony meatus. Secondary infection of this desquamated ball will cause a chronic discharge. Expansion of the deep bony canal is the diagnostic feature (Figure 9.25).

CLINICAL TESTS OF HEARING

Patients presenting with an otological complaint require their hearing to be assessed. Initially this is done by free-field speech testing followed by pure tone audiometry if an impairment is suspected.

FREE-FIELD SPEECH TEST

The prime object of free-field speech testing is to screen for the presence of a hearing impairment. Each ear is tested separately whilst masking the non-test ear. This is necessary because speech presented to the ear on one side of the head can be heard almost as easily by the other ear. Masking clinically is most easily done by pressing on the tragus with a finger and occluding the external auditory canal. A continuous sound is then created by constantly rubbing the tragus.

A normal hearing ear will hear a whispered voice at 360 cm (12 ft). A hearing impaired ear will be unable to hear a whispered voice at 60 cm (2 ft). The subject is instructed to repeat the words that are said to them and it is usual to test the better hearing ear first if there is one. Having ensured that the subject understands the task, lipreading is prevented by the examiner standing as far as possible behind the patient on the side of the test ear whilst masking the non-test ear with one hand. In order to ensure the use of a whispered voice, the inexperienced tester should exhale completely before whispering. What words are used is irrelevant provided they are not reused. A combination of numbers and letters such as '6D2' and 'C5H' prevents the examiner running out of words such as 'cookbook'. If the subject cannot repeat words spoken in a whisper at arm's length (60 cm, 2 ft) from the test ear then that ear is impaired.

FREE-FIELD VOICE TEST – SPECIALIST

The specialist, if sufficiently practised, can ascertain the degree of impairment with accuracy. Having identified that an impairment is present, the object is to assess the minimum voice level at which the subject can comprehend speech. There are two test positions, arm's length (60 cm, 2 ft) and as close to the ear as the tester may wish to speak (15 cm, 6 in). Halfway positions are of no value. There are three voice levels, whispered, normal conversational and loud voice, in ascending order. Table 9.2 shows the progression of testing through a whispered voice at 60 cm, to a whisper at 15 cm, to a conversational voice at 60 cm, to a conversational voice at 15 cm, to a loud voice at 60 cm. The threshold of hearing is that at which the majority (greater than 50%) of the syllables are repeated correctly. Opposite each threshold in the table is the likely degree of impairment matched by the likely pure-tone audiometric average over 0.5, 1, 2 and 4 kHz. Whenever a loud voice is used, masking with tragal rubbing produces insufficient noise. A clockwork noise box (Barany) is required.

TUNING FORK TESTS

The most commonly used tuning fork tests are the Rinne and Weber tests. Of these the Rinne test is the more useful as it helps to determine whether the hearing impairment has a conductive component to it. The physiological basis of the test is that the normal ear hears sound via air better than sound conducted through the bone of the skull. However, when a conductive deafness is present, sound heard via air is impaired and the patient hears better by bone conduction. An air–bone gap of greater than 30 dB will be correctly detected 75% of the time by the Rinne test. The only situation where the

Table 9.2 *Thresholds of free-field speech test*

Voice level	Distance	Impairment	PTA dB
Whisper	60 cm	Not impaired	<25
Whisper	15 cm	Mild	25–40
Conversation	60 cm	Moderate	41–50
Conversation	15 cm	Moderate	51–70
Loud voice	60 cm	Severe	71+

PTA, pure tone average over 0.5, 1, 2 and 4 kHz. These figures are approximate.

Rinne test is of real value is when the tympanic membrane is normal and the subject has a hearing impairment. In these circumstances otosclerosis is a potential diagnosis and, if in the Rinne test the bone conduction is louder than the air conduction, then this is almost certainly the diagnosis. Unfortunately, if the air conduction is louder than the bone conduction, otosclerosis cannot be ruled out. When the tympanic membrane is abnormal there is almost certainly a conduction defect and the Rinne test adds nothing.

The Weber test is only potentially of value in individuals with asymmetrical hearing and normal tympanic membranes. If they are abnormal the most likely reason for the asymmetry is a conduction defect in one ear and audiometry is required. When the tympanic membranes are normal it is indeed important to decide whether the asymmetry is due to an otosclerotic conductive impairment in one ear or an asymmetric sensorineural impairment. The latter could be due to an acoustic neuroma. Unfortunately, the Weber test is non-interpretable or incorrect in about 50% of such cases.

The golden rule is that whenever it is important to assess a hearing impairment, pure tone audiometry, correctly carried out with masking, is essential.

REFERENCES

Browning, G.G. 1995: Aetiopathology of inflammatory conditions of the external and middle ear. In Scott-Brown's *Otolaryngology*, 6th Edn, Otology Volume, Oxford: Butterworth-Heinemann

Browning, G.G. and Gatehouse, S. 1992: The prevalence of middle ear disease in the adult British population. *Clinical Otolaryngology* **17** 317–321.

Browning, G.G., Gatehouse, S. and Swan, I.R.C. 1991: The Glasgow benefit plot: A new method for reporting benefits from middle ear surgery. *Laryngoscope* **101**(2) 180–185.

Diamant, M. 1982: Mastoid pneumatization and cholesteatoma – the genetic question. In Sadé, J. (ed.) *Cholesteatoma and Mastoid Surgery. Proceedings of the 11th International Conference*, 105–110.

Effective Health Care 1992: *The treatment of persistent glue ear in children.* Department of Health Bulletin No. 4. London: HMSO.

McCormack, B. 1988: *Screening for hearing impairment in young children.* London: Croom Helm.

Sadé, J. and Berco, E. 1976: The atelectatic ears and secretory otitis media. *Annals of Otology Rhinology & Laryngology* Suppl. 25 166–72.

Tos, M., Stangerup, S.E. and Larsen, P. 1987: Dynamics of eardrum changes folowing secretory otitis. *Archives of Otolaryngology Head & Neck Surgery* **113** 380–385.

Wormald, P.J., Browning, G.G. and Robinson, K. 1995: Is otoscopy reliable? A structured teaching method to improve otoscopic accuracy in trainees. *Clinical Otolaryngology* **20** 63–67.

INDEX

Acute otitis media 10–11, 44–6
Attic cholesteatoma 63–4
Attico-antrostomy 66
Atticotomy 65
Aural toilet 82–6
  microsuction 85–6
  specialist 84–6

Barotrauma 75–6
Boils 50
Bullous myringitis 50, 51

Chalk patches 12, 35
Children
  hearing impairment 29–41
    otalgia 42–7
Cholesteatoma *see* Otitis media, chronic active
  squamous
Chronic otitis media *see* Otitis media, chronic
Cotton wool bud 83–4

Decision (summary) trees 2
  discharging ear (7.1) 53
  discharging ear – specialist (7.2) 58
  hearing impairment in adults (4.1) 18
  hearing impairment in children (5.1) 30
  layout of decision trees (1.1) 2
  otalgia in children (6.1) 44
  otalgia in adults (6.2) 47
  steps in otoscopy (2.1) 4
Discharging ear 52–74
  active chronic otitis media 54–73
  otitis externa 52–4

Ear, normal stucture 3–9
Epithelial pearl 69, 71, 77
Eustachian tube function 47

Examination techniques 78–88
Exostoses 86–7
External auditory canal 4–5
External ear, nerve supply 42

Foreign bodies 43
Free-field voice testing 31–2, 87–8
Furuncles 50

Glomus tumours 25–6
Granular myringitis 73
Grommets *see* Ventilating tubes

Hearing impairment
  adults 17–28
    summaries 26
  children 29–41
Healed otitis media 12, 24–5
Herpes zoster oticus 50, 51
Hopkins rod otoscope 81–2

Incisions 78–9
Inclusion cyst 77
Instruments, for otoscopy 78, 81–2

Keratosis obturans 87

Mastoid cavity disease *see also* Mastoidectomy
  discharging ear 55–6
  management 56, 72–3
  revision surgery 72–3
Mastoid obliteration 72
Mastoidectomy, modified radical 55–6, 66–73
  active 69–72
  active mucosal 70–1
  active squamosal 71
  inactive 66–8
  revision surgery 72–3
Mastoiditis, acute 46–7

Meatoplasty 55, 72
Microsuction 85–6
Middle ear
    carcinoma 73–4
    nerve supply 42
Middle ear pressure, negative 47
Modified radical mastoidectomy *see*
        Mastoidectomy
Myringitis
    bullous 50, 51
    granular 73

Negative middle ear pressure 47
Nerve supply, middle and external ear 42
Normal ear 3–9

Ossicular chain
    in chronic otitis media 20–3
    in negative middle ear pressure 47
    in otitis media with effusion 30
Otalgia 42–51
    adults 47–51
    causes 43
    children 42–7
    non-otologic 51
Otitis externa 5, 10, 43, 48–50
    benign necrotising 74
    malignant 49–50
    management 48–9
    specialist 49–50
Otitis media, healed 12, 24–5
Otitis media, acute 10–11, 44–6
Otitis media, chronic 8, 12–16
    active 54–60
    active mucosal 13, 14, 59, 60–1
    active squamous (cholesteatoma) 13, 14–15,
        61–5
        recurrent pearls 69, 71
    inactive, specialist 17–19
    inactive mucosal 15–16, 17–22
    inactive squamous (retractions) 16, 35–41
Otitis media, with effusion 11, 23–4, 30–41
    otological complications 35–41
    pain in 51
Otosclerosis 16, 27
Otoscopy 78–9
    limitations 80–1
    pneumatic 79–80

Painful ear *see* Otalgia
Pars flaccida 4–5, 6–9
    in chronic otitis media 12–16
    in active squamous chronic otitis media 63–5

Pars flaccida (*cont.*)
    retraction 8, 16, 38–41
        classification 39
Pars tensa 4–5, 6–9
    in active mucosal chronic otitis media 60–1
    in active squamous chronic otitis media 61–3
    in chronic otitis media 12–16
    number of quadrants 19
    retraction 8, 16, 35–8
        classification 36–8
    scarring 9
    traumatic perforation 76
    tympanosclerosis 12, 22, 35
Perforation *see* Pars tensa in chronic otitis media;
        Tympanic membrane
Pressure trauma 75–6
Prussack's space 38–9

Radionecrosis 74
Red ear, in acute otitis media 44–6
Rinne test 88
Rod otoscope 81–2

Schrapnell's membrane 6
Self trauma 75
Sensorineural hearing impairment
    asymmetrical 28
    children 29–30
    symmetrical 27
    due to trauma 76–7
Specialist sections
    acute otitis media 46
    aural toilet 84–6
    carcinoma of middle ear 73
    chronic otitis media 14–16
        active 57–73
        inactive 17–22
    discharging ear 57–73
    free-field voice testing 88
    healed otitis media 24–5
    glomus tumours 25–6
    granular myringitis 73
    otitis externa 49–50
    otitis media with effusion 23–4, 33–5
    retraction
        of pars flaccida 38–41
        of pars tensa 36–8
Speculum 80
Surgery
    mastoid cavity disease 72–3
Syringing
    trauma 75
    see also Aural toilet

Temporal bone
  fracture 76–7
  radionecrosis 74
Trauma
  pressure trauma 75–6
  self trauma 75
  surgical 76–7
Tuning fork tests 88
Tympanic membrane *see also* Pars tensa; Pars
    flaccida
  flush 84
  mobility in acute otitis media 46
    in pneumatic otoscopy 79–80
  normal 4–5, 6–9
  perforation
    marginal or central 18–20, 21

Tympanic membrane (*cont.*)
  perforation (*cont.*)
    site 17–20
    size 20
    traumatic 75–6
  routes of epithelial migration 4
  scars 9
Tympanosclerosis 12, 22, 35

Ventilating tubes (grommets) 33–4
  long term 23–4
Voice testing, free-field
  in children 31–2

Wax 4–5, 82–4
Weber test 88

INDEX OF PHOTOGRAPHS

Acute otitis media *2.19, 3.2, 6.3–6.6*
Barotrauma *8.3*
Bullous myringitis *6.16*
Carcinoma of ear *7.56*
Exostosis of canal *9.22–9.24*
Foreign body in canal *6.2*
Furuncle of canal *6.14*
Glomus tympanicum *4.23*
Glomus jugulare *4.24*
Granular myringitis *7.54–7.55*
Herpes zoster *6.15*
Healed otitis media *2.18, 3.4–3.5, 4.21–4.22,
    5.15–5.17*
Inclusion cyst *8.2*
Keratoma of canal *9.25*
Negative middle ear pressure *6.7*
Normal ear *2.5, 2.7, 2.9–2.14*
Otitis externa *2.6, 3.1, 6.8–6.10, 7.1–7.3*
    benign necrotising *7.58*
    fungal *6.11–6.12*
    malignant *6.13*
Otitis media – acute *2.19, 3.2, 6.3–6.6*
Otitis media – chronic
    active mucosal *3.7, 3.10–3.12, 4.11–4.12, 7.4–7.5,
        7.14–7.16, 7.18–7.23*

active mucosal with modified radical
    mastoidectomy *7.9–7.13, 7.42–7.46, 7.52*
active squamous (cholesteatoma) *3.8, 3.13–3.14,
    7.6–7.7, 7.24–7.30, 7.32–7.33*
active squamous (cholesteatoma) with modified
    radical mastoidectomy *7.47–7.50*
with atticotomy and attico-antrostomy *7.34–7.38*
inactive with modified radical mastoidectomy
    7.39–7.40, 7.52
inactive mucosal *2.15–2.16, 3.6, 3.9, 4.1–4.9,
    4.13–4.17, 7.17*
inactive squamous (retractions) *3.15–3.16,
    5.18–5.20, 5.22–5.28, 5.31–5.35, 7.31*
Otitis media with effusion *2.17, 2.20, 3.3, 4.18,
    5.2–5.10*
Otitis media, healed *2.18, 3.4–3.5, 4.21–4.22,
    5.15–5.16*
Otosclerosis *3.17, 4.25*
Radionecrosis *7.57*
Temporal bone fracture *8.5–8.6*
Trauma to canal *8.1–8.2*
Traumatic perforation *8.4*
Ventilating tubes (grommets) *4.19–4.20, 5.11–5.14*
Wax *2.3–2.4, 9.12–9.14*